BUILDING HEALTHY COMMUNITIES THROUGH MEDICAL-RELIGIOUS PARTNERSHIPS

BUILDING HEALTHY COMMUNITIES THROUGH MEDICAL-RELIGIOUS PARTNERSHIPS

SECOND EDITION

RICHARD G. BENNETT, M.D.
Raymond and Anna Lublin Professor in Geriatric Medicine
Johns Hopkins University School of Medicine
President, Johns Hopkins Bayview Medical Center
Baltimore, Maryland

and

W. DANIEL HALE, PH.D.
Professor of Psychology
Director, Community Health Initiative
Stetson University
DeLand, Florida
Adjunct Associate Professor of Medicine
Johns Hopkins University School of Medicine
Baltimore, Maryland

THE JOHNS HOPKINS UNIVERSITY PRESS
Baltimore

The Johns Hopkins University Press
2715 North Charles Street
Baltimore, Maryland 21218-4363
www.press.jhu.edu

Library of Congress Cataloging-in-Publication Data

Bennett, Richard G. (Richard Gordon)
Building healthy communities through medical-religious partnerships /
Richard G. Bennett and W. Daniel Hale. — 2nd ed.
     p. ; cm.
Rev. ed. of: Building healthy communities through medical-religious partnerships /
W. Daniel Hale and Richard G. Bennett. 2000.
Includes bibliographical references and index.
ISBN-13: 978-0-8018-9293-6 (pbk. : alk. paper)
ISBN-10: 0-8018-9293-7 (pbk. : alk. paper)
1. Community health services for older people—Religious aspects. 2. Managed care
plans (Medical care)—Religious aspects. 3. Older people—Medical care—Religious
aspects. 4. Preventive health services for older people—Religious aspects.
I. Hale, W. Daniel (William Daniel), 1950– II. Hale, W. Daniel (William Daniel),
1950– Building healthy communities through medical-religious partnerships. III. Title.
[DNLM: 1. Community Health Services—organization & administration. 2. Community-
Institutional Relations. 3. Health Education. 4. Patient Advocacy.
5. Religion and Medicine. WA 546.1 B472b 2009]
RA564.8.H35 2009
362.1′0425—dc22
2008042168

A catalog record for this book is available from the British Library.

*Special discounts are available for bulk purchases of this book. For more information, please
contact Special Sales at 410-516-6936 or specialsales@press.jhu.edu.*

To our parents

Wilford and Evelyn Bennett

William and Frances Hale

CONTENTS

FOREWORD

With health care reform in the air, this is the perfect time for this book, which describes creative models of how to make health care available through medical-religious partnerships. It explains how these partnerships can work by an interdisciplinary approach modeled in the book itself. Its organization by major illnesses, with information on each disease, highlights its medical perspective, which is rare for this genre of books. Extensive resources, including agencies and books on each illness, help provide the information needed to develop effective collaborative models.

Recent scientific studies have demonstrated the major role that religion can play in good health outcomes. In addition, patients and physicians are recognizing the importance of spiritual resources in the prevention of and recovery from illness. Congregations are seeing an expanding role in health care. A 2007 National Council of Churches survey of 6,000 congregations reported that 70 percent are engaged in health ministry. This favorable response is echoed by the authors' studies of various denominations.

The changing face of illness in the United States, from infectious diseases to more chronic illness plus the graying of our population, means that congregational support and educational programs are a key resource for long-term care needs as well as prevention strategies. The chapters on diabetes, dementia, mental illness, etc., specifically illustrate the congregation's role in addressing these and other illnesses.

Providing accurate, clear, and accessible health information is only one step to prevention. Motivating people to act on it is difficult, and congregations can be outstanding partners in that regard. Illustrative and effective programs, some of which have received large grants, encourage others to undertake such ministry, which can help reduce the $2.4 trillion annual expenditures in the United States as well as reduce the number of uninsured Americans, now at almost 46 million (2007 figures).

Some churches cannot undertake major programs, so the authors' suggestions for modest projects—such as training patient advocates and offering respite care programs, screenings, support groups, and informational mailings—enable almost any congregation to become involved in meeting health care needs. One creative program for church members was a "living wills party," hosted by a registered nurse in her home, which provided information and encouraged people to fill out an advance directive.

There is a particular need for destigmatization of mental illness, which affects members of religious communities and their families in about the same proportion—that is, 30 percent—as the general population. In this book we find clear, unbiased information with specifics on congregational approaches to mental illness, including ways for encouraging open sharing about personal mental health issues.

In addition to the chapters on disease, there are practical ones on advance directives and communicating with health care providers, a subject that touches many people. The section on lifestyle-related problems, addressed by exercise and diet, tobacco-cessation programs, etc., is brilliant, as all objections are answered with practical suggestions.

This book is a resource for lay people, health care professionals, pastors, community agency staff, and many others who are committed to meeting the health-related needs of all people.

The Rev. Dr. Abigail Rian Evans
Charlotte W. Newcombe Professor of Practical Theology
Princeton Theological Seminary

PREFACE

We prepared the original edition of *Building Healthy Communities through Medical-Religious Partnerships* because experience convinced us that partnerships between health care systems and religious congregations had tremendous potential to meet many of the difficult challenges our country faces as the population continues to age and the number of people with chronic conditions continues to increase. We had witnessed enthusiastic clergy, parish nurses, and congregational volunteers, supported by dedicated medical professionals, offering programs that helped people maintain their health, independence, and dignity. Almost a decade later, we are even more convinced of the valuable role that medical-religious partnerships can play in addressing the health needs of communities throughout our nation. The challenges described in the original volume are even greater now, and the models and resources that can be studied and employed by those interested in developing these partnerships have multiplied.

People who share our belief that health care systems, medical professionals, and religious congregations should join forces to minister to the health needs of their community will find in this book not only strong support for their belief but also detailed information and advice on programs that have proven successful in a diverse group of congregations and communities over the past decade. We report on innovative medical-religious partnership programs organized by Baptist, Catholic, Methodist, and Seventh Day Adventist health systems, along with other programs initiated and supported by health systems that have no current or historical ties to a national or local religious organization. We share stories of health programs offered by congregations representing a wide range of faiths and denominations (e.g., African Methodist Episcopal, Baptist, Catholic, Christian and

Missionary Alliance, Episcopal, Jewish, Lutheran, Methodist, Presbyterian, and Seventh Day Adventist) and from various parts of the country.

The introduction provides an overview of some of the most serious health challenges our country faces and why partnerships between health care systems and religious congregations are able to address these challenges. Clergy and lay leaders interested in seeing how a health program can complement existing ministries and programs will find an outstanding example in chapter 1, where we report on a congregational health program that has been going strong for more than 13 years. This program, coordinated entirely by volunteers, also illustrates how an effective and vibrant congregational health ministry can be run at virtually no expense to the church.

Health care professionals and religious leaders who have questions—and perhaps even some doubts—about the amount of interest in congregational health programs among parishioners and the types of program they believe are needed will find answers to many of these questions in the survey results reported in chapter 2. Elsewhere in that chapter we present a brief summary of the basic principles and methods of preventive medicine and illustrate how they can be incorporated into congregational programs. Chapter 3 provides an overview of the strategies that congregations can employ to link people with valuable health information and resources through proactive health education programs.

Part II focuses on specific chronic diseases and medical topics. Assisted by a panel of distinguished medical experts from the Johns Hopkins Medical Institutions, we provide, in a concise format designed specifically for individuals with little or no background in health care, the latest information about the most common diseases and the treatments for them. Each chapter includes suggestions for congregational programs and examples of such programs, and at the end of each chapter we provide information on additional resources.

In this section we also present strategies and resources that individuals can use to reduce their risk of illness and injury, effectively manage their medical conditions and health care, and maintain functional independence. Topics covered include lifestyle modifications, medication management, home safety, and advance directives. A chapter on communicating with health care providers includes a section on the concept of a patient advocacy or health partners program. This program trains individuals within a congregation to assist members with chronic illnesses who may not have relatives or close friends to help them navigate a complex health care system. Several of the chapters in this section include brief guides that can be reproduced and shared with interested persons. These guides are also available in PDF format on the Web site of the O'Neill Foundation for Community Health (www.oneillcommunityhealth.org) and can be downloaded and copied.

Finally, Part III provides up-to-date information on models that can be studied and resources that can be used by any individual or organization interested in developing medical-religious partnerships. Included is information on how to identify and access local agencies and organizations, along with descriptions and contact information for national organizations that offer valuable health education materials. Also included are descriptions of five different medical-religious partnership models, along with contact information for those who would like to learn more about the programs.

The programs and materials presented in this book are by no means exhaustive. Religious congregations can sponsor many other programs, and religious and medical institutions can work together in a number of different ways to enhance community health. There has never been a better time to explore innovative and collaborative efforts to minister to the health needs of communities. We are in the midst of a fundamental change in the way people are conceptualizing and organizing health care. Health care leaders are awakening to the fact that they need to reach out to the community through trusted institutions, and religious leaders are learning that they can ask for assistance and support from medical institutions. We encourage you to take the initiative to bring medical and religious communities closer together.

ACKNOWLEDGMENTS

We could not have written a book about community health partnerships without the assistance and goodwill of many people. First and foremost, we want to express our appreciation for the steadfast support and encouragement of the late Mr. and Mrs. William E. O'Neill. The programs we initially designed more than fifteen years ago could easily have gone no farther than the idea stage if it were not for their generosity and efforts on our behalf. Firmly convinced of the value of programs in which medical institutions and professionals worked in partnership with faith communities, they established a charitable foundation that continues to provide support for these programs. We are also indebted to their daughter, Mary O'Neill-Clement, the other members of the O'Neill family, and the individuals who have served as officers of the O'Neill Foundation for Community Health—Barbara Pearson; Bette Heins, Ph.D.; Bill Allen, J.D., M. Div.; and Lisa Ford Williams—for their continued support.

A number of health care leaders who have worked directly with us in key roles as we developed and implemented our programs deserve recognition for their contributions. These include Gail Camputaro (Volusia County Council on Aging); Tom Coleman, M.D. (Volusia County Health Department); Fran Davis (Hospice of Volusia/Flagler); Bill Griffin and Jeff Feasel (Halifax Health); Joe Johnson (Florida Hospital Fish Memorial); Mark LaRose and Mike Gentry (Florida Hospital Memorial Division); Daryl Tol (Florida Hospital DeLand); and Bob Williams (Bert Fish Medical Center). We are also grateful for the support and encouragement provided by Richard Kindred, Ph.D., and Grady Ballenger, Ph.D. (Stetson University).

We want to acknowledge the contributions of several individuals who have played important leadership roles in innovative faith-health partnerships and who offered to share their stories. Sonja Simpson, a faith community nurse and former president of the Health Ministries Association, not only wrote about her own work but also helped us identify other nurses who had similar stories to report. One of these individuals, Fran Zoske, wrote about many of the programs offered by hospitals affiliated with Ascension Health and contacted other faith community nurses who in turn shared their stories. We also greatly appreciate the contributions of Gary Gunderson, D. Min., who wrote about the programs he helped to develop for Methodist LeBonheur Healthcare in Memphis; Dale Young, D. Min., who shared his work developing the Congregational Health Alliance Ministry Program for Baptist Health South Florida; and Candace Huber, who reported on her work as director of Florida Hospital's Center for Community Health Ministry based in Orlando.

We would especially like to thank the Johns Hopkins faculty and staff who contributed to this edition by helping us update, revise, and improve the clinical chapters:

L. Randol Barker, M.D., Professor of Medicine, Johns Hopkins University School of Medicine

Kevin Bertha, R.Ph., Assistant Director of Pharmacy, Johns Hopkins Bayview Medical Center

Ilene Browner, M.D., Instructor in Medical Oncology, Johns Hopkins University School of Medicine

Thomas E. Finucane, M.D., Professor of Medicine, Johns Hopkins University School of Medicine

Linda Gorman, M.L.S., Director of Library Services, Johns Hopkins Bayview Medical Center

Sheldon H. Gottlieb, M.D., FACC, Associate Professor of Medicine, Johns Hopkins University School of Medicine

Steven Kravet, M.D., M.B.A., FACP, Assistant Professor of Medicine, Johns Hopkins University School of Medicine

Constantine G. Lyketsos, M.D., M.H.S., The Elizabeth Plank Althouse Professor in Alzheimer's Disease Research, Johns Hopkins University School of Medicine

Peter V. Rabins, M.D., M.P.H., Professor of Psychiatry, Johns Hopkins University School of Medicine

Annabelle Rodriguez-Oquendo, M.D., Associate Professor of Medicine, Johns Hopkins University School of Medicine

Jonathan M. Zenilman, M.D., Professor of Medicine, Johns Hopkins University School of Medicine

Susan Zieman, M.D., Ph.D., FACC, Assistant Professor of Medicine, Johns Hopkins University School of Medicine

Richard Zorowitz, M.D., Visiting Associate Professor of Physical Medicine and Rehabilitation, Johns Hopkins University School of Medicine

The expertise they brought to this work has made for a better book, for which we are most appreciative. Finally, we thank our editor, Wendy Harris, for her encouragement and guidance.

INTRODUCTION

Dramatic changes in American society are creating serious challenges for our health care systems, which evolved to treat acute illnesses but increasingly must adapt to care for chronic conditions. The most significant driver of this change is the aging of the population, a demographic trend that is accelerating. Current estimates are that more than 133 million Americans live with at least one chronic condition and that approximately half of these have multiple chronic conditions (Anderson 2007). As this group increases to almost 160 million by 2020 and more than 170 million by 2030 (Anderson 2007), the impact of these chronic diseases will be felt in many ways. These illnesses are the leading cause of mortality, accounting for seven out of every ten deaths (Partnership to Fight Chronic Disease 2008). People with chronic conditions are responsible for more than 90 percent of all prescription drugs used, more than 80 percent of all inpatient hospital stays, more than 75 percent of all visits to physicians, and approximately 85 percent of all health care expenditures (Anderson 2007).

What is often obscured by statistics such as these, and what makes chronic diseases so challenging, is that much of the care for people with chronic diseases is provided, not in hospitals or physicians' offices, but in the homes of the affected individuals. And most of that care is provided, not by physicians and nurses, but by the individuals themselves. Medical professionals and institutions continue to play essential roles with respect to chronic diseases, particularly for acute exacerbations, but the responsibility for the day-to-day management of most of these diseases—monitoring the conditions, using medications correctly, implementing and then sustaining recommended lifestyle modifications—rests largely with the affected individuals themselves or those who assist them at home in their care. Thus, health care organizations committed to improving the health of their communities must find ways to reach out to those who have chronic diseases and others who are at risk for chronic diseases and to provide them with the information and support they need to manage their conditions and to use medical services in a timely and appropriate manner.

Another serious challenge facing health care systems is the increasing ethnic and racial diversity of their communities. It is expected that by 2010 minority ethnic and racial groups will make up 35 percent of the U.S. population and that by 2020 this number will increase to almost 39 percent (U.S. Census Bureau 2004). At the same time that we are becoming more diverse, the health status of most racial and ethnic minorities continues to lag behind that of the rest of the population (U.S. Department of Health and Human Services 2000, 2006). Increasingly, health care systems will have to develop programs that are responsive to the special medical needs of various minority groups and that reflect an understanding of the values and traditions of these groups. Clinicians working with minorities will need to pay special attention to the issue of trust because mistrust of medical institutions and professionals can be a significant barrier to the delivery of needed services.

So how can health care organizations, most of which are experiencing severe financial pressures, address these challenges? Where can they find the resources to educate large numbers of people about chronic diseases? How can they reach the people in their community who have no ties to the health care system and are not even aware that they may have a chronic condition? How can they tailor programs to meet the needs of increasingly diverse communities? And how can they overcome the mistrust of medical institutions that exists among some groups?

There is a way for health care organizations, large and small, to address these challenges. But they cannot do it by themselves. To reach and maintain contact with people, providing them with the information and resources they need to make good decisions about their health and medical care, health care organizations need partners. They need to work closely with institutions that are deeply rooted in the community and are trusted by people in the community. Health care organizations need to develop alliances with institutions that have a strong tradition of caring for others and that attract people who identify with this tradition.

Religious congregations—churches, synagogues, mosques, and temples—clearly fit this description. They have the community resources and communication networks that hospitals need. Just as important, they have the altruistic traditions and values that are at the heart of community-based health programs. No community institutions are better suited to serve as partners for hospitals. This is especially true for addressing the health needs of older adults and families who have the responsibility of caring for older adults. Whereas most children and adolescents can be reached through school-based health promotion programs and most young and middle-aged adults can be reached through work-site initiatives, religious institutions are the one place where large numbers of older adults regularly gather.

Over the last fifteen years, we have witnessed the tremendous impact that medical-religious partnerships can have on the health of communities, reaching large numbers of people who had not been reached by other health programs. We have seen enthusiastic nurses and volunteers from religious congregations work closely with health care organizations and medical professionals to organize programs focusing on the management of specific diseases, such as high blood pressure and diabetes. Through such programs, participants have been alerted to the need to identify these conditions as early as possible to minimize future complications. Some programs have helped people recognize and respond promptly to the earliest signs of a heart attack or stroke, and other programs have instructed people how to use advance directives to maintain control over their medical care if they become incapacitated due to injury or illness. Valuable information about hospice care has been presented by health professionals and reinforced by clergy. Reminders about screenings and vaccinations and information about where these services are available have been printed in congregational bulletins and announced during worship services and other congregational gatherings. Through programs like these—programs that have brought together the expertise and resources of the medical community with the dedication and energy of volunteers from religious congregations—people have become more knowledgeable about important medical issues and the medical services available in their communities as well as more skillful in working with their own physicians and other health care providers.

We have been particularly impressed with the effectiveness of medical-religious partnerships in reaching minority communities. When health care organizations have demonstrated a sincere interest in working with members of predominately minority congregations to address their concerns in a culturally sensitive fashion, this interest has been met with enthusiastic support from clergy and lay leaders. They have welcomed representatives of health care organizations to their communities and offered valuable advice about how to break down barriers that have kept many from receiving health services.

One of the encouraging aspects of programs built around medical-religious partnerships, and one of the reasons they have great potential to address some of the most serious health care challenges of the twenty-first century, is how much can be accomplished without straining the financial resources of health care organizations. Most hospitals and medical centers already have the materials, services, and personnel needed to offer programs to religious congregations. They do not need to create new departments or hire additional personnel.

Believing as strongly as we do in the need for communities throughout the country to forge medical-religious partnerships, we have prepared a book that can be used to introduce the basic idea of these partnerships to medical and religious leaders—to help them "catch the vision" and to serve as a manual or guide for health programs. In writing this book, we have drawn not only on our own experience but also on that of hospital administrators, physicians, nurses, clergy, and congregational volunteers who have been involved in medical-religious partnerships in many different communities.

Health care systems can begin building partnerships with congregations in several ways. Most hospitals already have a broad network of contacts with the religious leaders of their own communities, and these local clergy regularly provide pastoral care for inpatients or serve on ethics committees. Many larger hospitals employ full- or part-time religious professionals who become active members of the health care team and typically provide oversight and management for the hospitals' volunteer clergy staff. These individuals can be engaged to begin an outreach program designed to strengthen ties between the single hospital and the multiple faith communities that typically surround it. Inaugural programs can be structured as evening seminars that provide an overview of the contents of this book and review the resources that the hospital can make available to interested congregations. Alternatively, a wider net can be cast, and copies of the book can be sent to local congregations with a letter directing interested recipients to call for more information.

Special attention and efforts may be needed when hospitals seek to establish relationships with congregations in parts of the community where members may be doubtful or even suspicious about the motives behind a hospital's new outreach program. In these situations, it is advisable to make direct contact with a telephone call and an offer to visit clergy and lay leaders at their own local house of worship to describe this opportunity more fully and to begin building a trusting relationship that can serve as the foundation for programs that will empower all members of the community to better care for themselves, their families, and their neighbors.

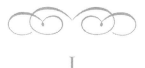

I

THE RELIGIOUS CONGREGATION
AND HEALTH CARE

1

HEALING BODY, MIND, AND SOUL—
A MODEL FOR HEALTH MINISTRY

Rev. Jeffrey Sumner had approached the summer of 1999 full of optimism and enthusiasm as he worked with members of the congregation to prepare for Vacation Bible School and various other summer programs. He had no reason to think that he might have a serious medical condition. As far as he could tell, he was in excellent health, and everything seemed to be going well at church and at home. Although his first few years at Westminster by-the-Sea Presbyterian Church in Daytona Beach, Florida, had been stressful as he helped the congregation heal the deep wounds and divisions that had occurred prior to his arrival, the last few years had been especially gratifying. The congregation had doubled in size during his tenure and now offered ministries and programs that drew people of all ages. Sunday morning worship services were well attended, Sunday school classrooms were full, and so many young families had joined the church that the nursery had been expanded to three rooms. It wasn't just on Sundays that people came to the church. Almost every day the buildings were buzzing with activity. Life was good at home too. There were no unusual or particularly difficult stresses. In fact, his wife, Mary Ann, and their three children all seemed to be thriving. He could look at his family and his work with a great deal of satisfaction. Life was indeed good!

Feeling as well as he did physically and emotionally, Rev. Sumner could easily have gone several more years without discovering he had a serious medical problem had he not stopped by the church fellowship hall on that morning in June to participate in a health screening. This screening, open to the wider community as well as to members of the congregation, was offered as part of Body, Mind, and Soul, the health ministry developed in collaboration with a local hospital and led by volunteers from his congregation. Fortunately, he did attend the screening, though his primary motivation was simply to show support for the program. And even then he almost escaped testing. His busy schedule had kept him from being present at the beginning of the screenings, so by the time he arrived, all of the risk assessment forms had been used. He graciously offered to forgo the testing because he was certain he did not have any health problems, but the nurse coordinating the program insisted that she go to her car to get a form for him. She felt that it was important for him, as a congregational leader, to go through the screening.

After giving him time to complete the risk assessment form, the nurse drew a small sample of his blood to be tested. But a few minutes later, instead of giving him the results, she told him that she needed to run the test again because the equipment might have malfunctioned. After the second test was completed, she reported back to him that she had encountered the same problem and wanted her supervisor to run a third test. Only after this third test was Rev. Sumner given the results, and they were not what he had expected. The nurse discreetly informed him that she was concerned about what she had found. Each of the three tests had shown a blood sugar level of over 350, well above what was considered normal. His cholesterol level also was abnormally high. While not conclusive, these results led her to suspect that he had diabetes. She then briefly explained what it meant to have diabetes and why it was important that he begin treatment as soon as possible if he had it. She strongly recommended that he see his family physician to have tests run that could yield a more certain diagnosis.

Rev. Sumner was in shock as he left the fellowship hall, numb from the news that he might have diabetes. How could this be? How could he feel so good and yet have a condition that could wreak havoc throughout his body? Wanting to know for sure if he had diabetes, he called his family physician and was able to schedule an appointment for later that day. Dr. Jennings agreed that diabetes seemed likely and ordered blood tests for the following morning that would be more conclusive. When the results came back, there was no more doubt about the diagnosis. Rev. Sumner had type 2 diabetes and would need to begin treatment immediately.

The treatment plan that Dr. Jennings outlined at Rev. Sumner's next appointment was different from what many patients expect from their physicians and what would have been recommended had Rev. Sumner been diagnosed with an infection or another acute illness. He was given a prescription for a medication that would help him control the diabetes, but Dr. Jennings made it clear that the medication would be only one part of the overall treatment regimen. There was no quick and easy fix for diabetes. It was a chronic condition that would always be a part of Rev. Sumner's life, and it would require his daily attention. His blood sugar would need to be checked three times a day, and he would be the person in charge of that monitoring. An effective treatment regimen would also include significant changes in diet and daily routines, and here again he would bear the responsibility for implementing and maintaining these changes.

Dr. Jennings supplemented his explanation of diabetes and his treatment recommendations with printed materials that explained in more detail just how important diet and exercise would be in controlling diabetes, but he knew that even these handouts would not provide all of the information Rev. Sumner would need or answer all of the questions that were sure to arise. For this reason, he strongly recommended that Rev. Sumner enroll in a course on diabetes offered by the hospital.

Heeding his doctor's advice, Rev. Sumner contacted the hospital, where he learned that he would be expected to bring Mary Ann with him to all of the classes. Although she did not have diabetes, it would be important for her to learn about the disease and what she could do to help him monitor and control it. Mary Ann, who had already purchased several books on diabetes for the family, readily agreed to join him.

One of the first things they learned from the course instructor, Chris Willman, was just how harmful diabetes could be if not brought under control. They learned about the many serious long-term complications that could develop, including blindness, heart disease, stroke, kidney failure, amputations, and nerve damage. Rev. Sumner was especially concerned about the risk of amputations and loss of vision. He could not imagine what it would be like to continue in his vocation if he were unable to read or to move about easily.

Although Ms. Willman wanted to impress on those attending the course the serious risks associated with diabetes, her purpose was not to scare them. Rather, her goal was to empower them by giving them the knowledge and skills they would need to gain control of their diabetes. She explained how the failure of their bodies to produce or appropriately use insulin resulted in abnormally high levels of glucose in the bloodstream that over time would do serious damage to various parts of their bodies. To avoid these damaging effects, they would need to monitor their blood glucose levels regularly and adopt eating habits and exercise routines that could keep their blood glucose levels in a safe range. She showed them how to check their blood sugar and then had them practice doing it. For those who needed insulin to control their diabetes, she explained how and when to take it. They learned what to eat, how much to eat, and when to eat. With her guidance, they discovered how to prepare meals that would be healthy as well as tasty. She also stressed the importance of regular physical activity and of establishing an exercise routine that fit their schedules and interests.

There was a lot to learn, but by the end of the course Rev. Sumner's anxiety about diabetes was largely gone, replaced by information that could be used to bring his diabetes under control. There was no question that his life was going to be different in many respects now that he had a chronic disease, but he emerged from the course convinced that his life would still be a full, active one as long as he took good care of himself.

Next came the real challenge for Rev. Sumner—translating his newly acquired knowledge about diabetes into a course of action. Because faithfully following treatment recommendations involves changing habits and routines that are firmly established and often highly pleasurable, this can be a difficult hurdle for patients with diabetes. What can make this even more challenging is that family members, co-workers, and friends may not understand and support their efforts. Fortunately, this was not the case for Rev. Sumner—at least not at home. After the initial shock of hearing that their father had diabetes, his children decided to educate themselves about his illness and do what they could to help him maintain his health. For example, as soon as they understood the important role diet played in controlling diabetes, they willingly joined with their father in preparing and eating healthier meals. And when they learned that their father had decided to begin a regular exercise routine of long walks in the neighborhood, they bought him a portable tape player (later upgraded to an iPod) so that he could listen to his favorite music along the way.

Rev. Sumner found that support and encouragement came from his church family as well. Thanks in large measure to the many health seminars and discussions held at the church, there was a spirit of openness and trust about medical issues among members of the congregation. They had become more comfortable discussing health concerns that previously they might have shared only with family members. Rev. Sumner had encouraged this openness, recognizing that speaking openly about a feared issue usually relieved much of the anxiety and frequently led to helpful suggestions and offers of help from others. Now it was his turn to share his medical concerns with members of the congregation and to ask for their understanding as he made certain changes in his life. He did this by writing the congregation a letter that he read to them before a Sunday worship service and subsequently printed in the church's monthly newsletter.

Members of the congregation, now aware of the medical challenges their minister faced, responded with kind words and deeds. Several who had diabetes shared their stories with him and offered encouragement. A teenage girl from church who had diabetes visited him to demonstrate how she measured her blood sugar and to talk about how she coped with diabetes. Her fearless and confident approach bolstered Rev. Sumner's confidence. The parishioners in charge of congregational meals began checking with him to make sure that at church dinners there were food choices that would allow him to stay on his diet. Members who invited Rev. Sumner into their homes for a meal did the same. Many members unobtrusively checked in with him from to time to time to be sure he was taking good care of himself.

By the end of the summer, Rev. Sumner, who as a Presbyterian minister was used to passionately sharing the gospel of Jesus Christ, found what he called his "second gospel": that through proper monitoring, awareness, and partnerships with physicians, people in congregations and communities can live longer and healthier lives when armed with knowledge and opportunities for healthy life choices.

As Rev. Sumner reflected on the experiences of the last few months, he realized just how important the church's Body, Mind, and Soul program had been to him and to so many others. Through the information and resources the program had brought into the congregation, he and the members of the church had learned valuable lessons that could help them prevent serious injuries and illnesses, detect diseases while they were at a treatable stage, manage chronic conditions, and find relief from many of the burdens of caregiving. Several of these lessons were clearly illustrated in his recent experiences.

Looking and feeling healthy does not necessarily mean that you are healthy. Just because he was free of pain and full of energy did not mean that he was free of disease. It had been easy for him to lull himself into a false sense of security about his health simply because he was feeling good.

Easy access to health screenings and preventive care can increase the use of these services. Like many people, his busy schedule often got in the way of proper preventive care. It had been much easier to stop by the church for a screening than it would have been to get to the lab at the hospital or an outpatient clinic.

Successful treatment for most chronic conditions requires patients to become well informed and actively engaged in their medical care. He had learned that he would bear the responsibility for the day-to-day monitoring and management of his diabetes, and to do so, he needed to become knowledgeable about the disease and its treatment.

Good medical care is built around a partnership between patients and their physicians that allows for the free flow of information in both directions. To provide an accurate diagnosis and effective treatment plan, his physician needed him to share all aspects of his life that might contribute to his condition or serve as barriers to effective treatment; and for the treatment to be successful, his physician needed to explain the diagnosis and treatment strategy in clear, understandable terms.

Coping with a chronic illness is easier when you are open with family and friends. The support, cooperation, and encouragement he had received from his family and the congregation made it easier to follow his doctor's treatment recommendations and to cope with the emotional dimension of diabetes.

BODY, MIND, AND SOUL

The health screening at which Rev. Sumner learned he had diabetes was just one part of Body, Mind, and Soul, the comprehensive health ministry at Westminster by-the-Sea Presbyterian Church. This popular ministry had grown out of an innovative community health education program sponsored by a nearby hospital. Hospital administrators and physicians at Halifax Health Medical Center had long recognized the need in their community for more education about disease prevention and illness management. Every day they saw people coming through their doors with serious medical problems that could have been averted if they had taken the right steps or at least sought treatment before the disease had reached an advanced stage. They saw others who had been properly diagnosed and received appropriate treatment initially but then failed, for one reason or another, to follow through with the treatment recommendations they had received. The hospital administrators and medical professionals knew they needed to find a way to reach out into the community with the information and resources that would enable people to maintain their health and to use the hospital and other medical services in a timely and appropriate way. They needed a systematic approach that provided stronger ties, more continuity, and greater support.

When hospital administrators and several key physicians learned of a successful community health education program in Baltimore that involved a medical center's reaching out into the community through religious congregations, they decided to develop a similar program in Daytona Beach and the surrounding communities. Their program, like the one in Baltimore, would rely largely on volunteers from congregations willing to be trained as "lay health educators." With guidance from physicians at the Johns Hopkins University School of Medicine, they created a curriculum focused primarily on common chronic conditions—hypertension, heart disease, cancer, diabetes, depression, and dementia. Course material included information on the prevalence of each of these conditions, the reasons they often went undetected, the risk of complications if these conditions went untreated, and the steps people could take to prevent or at least gain control over these conditions. They also covered medication management, influenza and pneumococcal vaccinations, prevention of accidents and falls, and advance directives. Once the curriculum was established, they had no trouble finding physicians, nurses, pharmacists, and other health providers affiliated with the hospital willing to serve as instructors and then provide ongoing support for volunteers as they developed their congregational programs.

With the curriculum and instructors in place, the next step was to recruit volunteers from local congregations. This was done by contacting clergy and inviting them to join with the hospital in developing congregational health programs. Those who were interested were asked to identify one or two members of their congregation who would be interested in being trained as lay health educators. It was explained that the program would give volunteers the information and tools they needed to coordinate health education seminars, screenings, and support groups in their congregation. They also would learn about the various medical services and be equipped to serve as liaisons between their congregation and the hospital.

Twenty-five volunteers participated the first time this course was offered, meeting at the hospital two hours each week for eight weeks. When the course was completed, there was enough interest among local congregations for the course to be offered twice more. By the end of the first year, 59 volunteers from religious congregations and retirement communities had completed training as lay health educators.

Nancy Force, the volunteer from Westminster by-the-Sea Presbyterian Church, was like most of her classmates in the lay health educator program in that she had no formal training or experience in health care. What she did have was good organizational skills, an eagerness to reach out to people in need, and experience caring for her late husband during the chemotherapy and surgeries he endured as he battled cancer. By the time she had completed the course, she was ready and eager to start organizing health programs in her congregation. Working closely with Rev. Sumner and members of her congregation and sometimes with members of nearby congregations, she developed a series of programs covering what she had learned during her training. The enthusiastic response of the congregation and community to these programs was truly gratifying. Programs were well attended, often drawing a third or more of the audience from outside the congregation.

Unlike some programs that are popular when first offered but then fade away over time or come to an end when the original leader leaves, Body, Mind, and Soul grew in popularity and had become such an integral part of the overall ministry of the church that when Nancy Force needed to step down as coordinator, there was no question that the program would continue. Tina Buck, an elder in the church who was employed at that time by a large health care organization, continued the program and added new topics. Later Helen Chandler, a nurse and elder in the congregation, took over and served as coordinator for several years. And when she left this position to head up another church program, Alexis Fortune stepped in and kept the program running strong.

Shortly after Body, Mind, and Soul celebrated its twelfth anniversary, Rev. Sumner sat down with me (WDH) to review the program's offerings and to discuss the many ways he felt the program had benefited members of the congregation and others from outside the church who had attended some of the offerings. He started by going over some of the topics that had been covered, summarizing the key points that had been emphasized by speakers and in the materials that often were handed out at seminars or included in congregational bulletins and newsletters.

Heart Disease. Rev. Sumner easily recalled a number of important points covered in the programs and materials devoted to heart disease. One was that heart disease remains the number one cause of death for women as well as for men, something that surprises many people. The importance of recognizing the earliest signs of a heart attack and then taking prompt action was stressed. Handouts listing warning signs of a heart attack were distributed and discussed, with attention being called to the fact that not all individuals experience crushing chest pain. As for prompt action, CPR instruction was arranged for one session, and people were advised to call 911 immediately rather than trying to drive themselves or a loved one to the hospital and also to take an aspirin while awaiting the paramedics' arrival. Programs and materials also emphasized that changes in lifestyle—particularly a low-fat diet, regular physical activity, and stopping smoking—along with careful monitoring and control of cholesterol and blood pressure, could greatly reduce their risk of a heart attack.

Stroke. As with heart disease, programs and materials placed an emphasis on early detection and quick action. People were encouraged to think of strokes as "brain attacks" requiring immediate care. Lists of warning signs were distributed and reviewed, and the role of high blood pressure as a major risk factor was stressed. Special note was made of the fact that people could have dangerously high blood pressure and not be aware of it—thus, the importance of having it checked regularly. Lifestyle factors that could increase the risk of stroke were also reviewed.

Cancer. When we came to the topic of cancer, Rev. Sumner reported that the emphasis on early detection, something underscored in almost all programs and materials on the topic, had a special meaning for the congregation. Within a period of less than eighteen months, two young men in the congregation, both in their thirties, had died of melanoma. Still feeling these tragic losses, members of the congregation were eager to learn about the methods for early detection of cancer, including colonoscopy, mammography, and breast self-examination. In seminars and the accompanying material, common misconceptions about these methods were directly addressed and corrected. And with respect to the prevention and early detection of skin cancer, the congregation not only spread the word among members but joined in sponsoring an annual community-wide event that raised awareness of the importance of screenings and also raised funds for a foundation that supported research on melanoma.

Diabetes. One of the major points emphasized in programs and materials was that in as many as one-third of adults with diabetes, the condition goes undetected and untreated. Coupled with this startling statistic was information about how untreated diabetes puts individuals at risk for a number of conditions that can cripple or kill, including heart disease and stroke. Symptoms that otherwise might be ignored, such as thirst, blurry vision, and fatigue, were listed, and the importance of maintaining a healthy diet and weight was emphasized.

Depression. One of the major goals of the programs on depression was to reduce the stigma that is still too often associated with mental illness. Rev. Sumner reinforced this message every chance he had, encouraging people to think of depression much as they think of other medical conditions and not as a sign of personal weakness. Another key point emphasized was that in most cases depression could be successfully treated through medication and/or psychotherapy, and that they should discuss their symptoms and concerns with their physician. Suggestions for recognizing symptoms and how to reach out to people who might be experiencing depression also were given. Counselors from their local Presbyterian Counseling Center took the lead in addressing this topic.

Dementia. Much of the information on dementia addressed the issue of the tremendous burden Alzheimer's disease and other forms of dementia can place on family caregivers, who may feel that it is their responsibility to provide all of the care for a loved one or who may be unaware of community agencies that offer various forms of assistance, including respite care.

Caregivers were urged to avail themselves of resources the church and other organizations offered. Also discussed was the value of having dementia diagnosed in its earliest stage because that allows patients to participate in the planning for their care during the later stages.

Palliative Care and Hospice. The programs on palliative care featured information on the services of local hospice organizations, with special attention given to common misconceptions about hospice care (e.g., that it is only for people who have cancer or AIDS, that it is only for the final days or weeks of life) that often interfere with the timely and appropriate use of these services. Another issue addressed was the importance of advance directives that allow individuals to maintain control of their care even if an injury or illness should prevent them from communicating their wishes. In addition to providing information about advance directives, the church keeps in the office a supply of the Five Wishes form developed by Aging with Dignity and gives members the option of having a copy of their completed form kept at the church.

Managing Medications. Advice and strategies for effective management of medications were offered at programs led by pharmacists and also as part of programs focusing on specific illnesses (e.g., heart disease, depression). A key point emphasized in all programs was that every physician a patient sees should be aware of every medication that patient is taking, including over-the-counter medications. Pharmacists and physicians also emphasized that patients should not discontinue a prescribed medication without first discussing the matter with their physician.

Home Safety. One of the key messages of programs on preventing falls and accidents was that individuals should not be reluctant to use assistive devices (e.g., canes, walkers, and wheelchairs) if they have a condition that increases their risk of falling. This message was reinforced by Rev. Sumner with individual members whenever he thought it might be appropriate and by the church's program of loaning walkers and wheelchairs to members. He even told those with walkers to think of them as their "everlasting arms" and to "lean on them" even when they felt self-conscious about using them. Other programs and materials on accident prevention and securing homes from intruders and scam artists provided advice and simple ways to make people's lives safer.

On-site Screenings. One of the key points emphasized in several of the educational seminars was that it is possible for people to be unaware that they have a potentially serious medical condition. Therefore, it is important for them to be screened for various conditions, even if they are experiencing no symptoms. To reinforce this point and to remove some of the obstacles that often get in the way of people scheduling screenings at their doctor's office or a hospital laboratory, Rev. Sumner and the leaders of Body, Mind, and Soul decided to arrange for screenings to be conducted at the church and, whenever possible, in conjunction with regularly scheduled services and programs. An excellent example of making a screening easily accessible is the church's program of screening for skin cancer. Participation in these screenings, conducted annually and offered immediately after the Sunday morning worship service by local dermatologists, is always high (50–90 individuals), and several members have discovered that they had a suspicious lesion that warranted further medical attention. Body, Mind, and Soul also arranges for blood pressure screenings and hearing tests to be conducted. These, like the skin cancer screenings, are offered immediately after the Sunday morning worship service during the church's fellowship hour when members and visitors mingle and enjoy light snacks. Body, Mind, and Soul also sponsors screenings for diabetes, like the one where Rev. Sumner first learned he had diabetes, and cardiac risk factors (i.e., cholesterol and triglycerides). These are done in coordination with the hospital's laboratory and typically offered on weekdays rather than Sunday.

On-site Preventive Care. With approximately half of the congregation in the age group most at risk for serious complications from influenza (65 years of age or older), the leaders of Body, Mind, and Soul decided they wanted to do more than educate members about the importance of vaccinations. Working with the county health department, they have arranged to offer vaccinations at the church every fall. Each year this is preceded by an educational campaign to inform members of the benefits of influenza vaccinations and to correct misconceptions about its dangers. A similar program for vaccination against pneumonia is offered at the church every other year.

Congregational Care Teams. This program, established following a presentation by a local hospice organization, brings together small groups of volunteers to provide non-medical care and support for individuals whose ability to live independently is threatened by their frailty or medical condition. A team's activities often include transportation, shopping, and light housework, with each team dividing up the workload so that no member is overwhelmed by caregiving responsibilities. Complementary congregational programs have also used speakers from the Council on Aging to describe sources for financial and physical assistance.

Support Groups. The church is home to Alcoholics Anonymous, Al-Anon, and Gamblers Anonymous support groups. Rev. Sumner noted that the church does more than provide meeting space for these support groups. In each case, there is at least one member of the congregation who, because of the openness and trust that exists among church members, has been willing to speak publicly about his or her struggles with an addiction and to encourage others who are also battling an addiction to seek help and support.

Exercise and Weight-Reduction Groups. Body, Mind, and Soul has hosted several programs demonstrating proper exercises for back pain and cardiovascular strengthening. In addition, the church now has a weekly "Meditation and Stretching" class to help people with their physical, emotional, and spiritual challenges. One of the serendipitous developments Rev. Sumner has witnessed is members, convinced of the health benefits of regular physical activity, finding others in the congregation who enjoy the same type of activity and want to have a partner or group to join with them. Similar pairings or groups have been formed among members interested in weight reduction.

As we neared the conclusion of our conversation, Rev. Sumner emphasized just how much this program means to the congregation. It is not simply the number of people attending seminars or participating in screenings that impresses him. It is also the conversations he hears among members as they gather for Sunday school classes or visit with each other during the fellowship hour. It is not unusual for them to be discussing their latest blood pressure readings or cholesterol levels or their plans for a colonoscopy or mammogram, and doing so with an informed understanding of these topics. Their church has come to be known not only as a reliable source of Christian teaching but also as a reliable source of health information.

The program's influence is also evidenced throughout the week in homes and doctors' offices and hospitals throughout the Daytona Beach area. People who have participated in the offerings of Body, Mind, and Soul carry with them a well-placed sense of confidence about health matters. Medical professionals and the health care system are no longer as intimidating as they once had been. These participants believe in the value of regular medical visits, and they know how to make the best use of the time with their doctors. They have a greater appreciation of the need to understand and follow the treatment recommendations of their physicians. They know what symptoms or physical sensations signal a call to 911 or a trip to the hospital's emergency department. Participants have a belief in their ability to reduce their risk of premature illness, disability, and death, and they act on this belief. They are eager to share what they have learned through these programs with family, friends, and colleagues. There is no doubt in Rev. Sumner's mind and in the minds of dozens of health professionals who have participated in the church's health ministry that this program, built around partnerships with health care organizations, continues to have a significant and far-reaching impact on the congregation and community.

2

ADDRESSING CHALLENGES THROUGH MEDICAL-RELIGIOUS PARTNERSHIPS

The Body, Mind, and Soul health ministry of Westminster by-the-Sea Presbyterian Church (chapter 1) is an example of how a religious congregation can effectively address serious health challenges by working in partnership with health care organizations, but it is only one of many such programs throughout the country. We have worked with congregations of all sizes and faiths, some in large cities and others in suburban communities and small towns. Despite differences in size and religious beliefs and practices, these congregations share several features that make them ideal partners for health care organizations interested in reaching out into the community.

One of the most important features is that houses of worship are the *only* place in our society where older adults, the age group with the greatest prevalence of chronic conditions, gather regularly in large numbers. The U.S. Religious Landscape Survey, a nationwide survey of a representative sample of more than 35,000 adults, found that 54 percent of adults in the 65 or older age group reported attending religious services at least once a week, with another 11 percent attending at least once or twice a month (Pew Forum on Religion and Public Life 2008). Another important feature, especially given the increasing diversity of the U.S. population, is that regular attendance is even higher among African American and Hispanic adults (Gallup and Newport 2006).

Religious congregations bring several other important aspects to partnerships with health care organizations:

- There are more than 330,000 religious congregations in the United States (*Yearbook of American and Canadian Churches, 2008*), or approximately 65 congregations for each of the country's 5,000 community hospitals (*Statistical Abstract of the United States, 2008*). These congregations are generally spread throughout the various neighborhoods of a community and thus are accessible and familiar to residents.

- Religious congregations are not only located in the community but also generally established and governed in large measure by residents of the community. Thus, they are likely to reflect the traditions and values of community residents and to be trusted as well.

- Most religious institutions have excellent facilities and equipment for educational programs, with ample parking and seating and a good sound system.

- Religious congregations generally have well-established communication networks that allow them to stay in touch with their members. Information can be disseminated by announcements during congregational gatherings, bulletins distributed at worship services, newsletters and other mailings sent to members at their home, Web sites, e-mails, and volunteer phone networks.

- Perhaps most important is the *human capital* found within religious congregations. This term embraces the rich human resources within most religious institutions. Churches, synagogues, and mosques have established traditions of volunteerism and civic engagement. In every congregation there are members, especially among those who are older, who are willing not only to volunteer their time but also to participate in congregational training programs that enhance their ability to step into leadership roles and to be of service to others in their congregations and communities. Many are retirees with rich experience able to bring incredible energy to a task.

These communication networks and volunteer activities usually reach well beyond the membership of a congregation. Robert Putnam, in his acclaimed analysis of American society *Bowling Alone: The Collapse and Revival of American Community,* describes faith communities as "arguably the single most important repository of social capital in America" (2000, 66). He cites a number of studies and surveys to support this claim. For example, "In one survey of twenty-two different types of voluntary associations, from hobby groups to professional associations to veterans groups to self-help groups to sports clubs to service clubs, it was membership in religious groups that was most closely associated with other forms of civic involvement, like voting, jury service, community projects, talking with neighbors, and giving to charity" (67). And he reports that "religiously involved people seem simply to know more people. One intriguing survey that asked people to enumerate all individuals with whom they had had a face-to-face conversation in the course of the day found that religious attendance was the most powerful predictor of the number of one's daily personal encounters. Regular church attendees reported talking with 40 percent more people in the course of the day" (67).

These features of religious congregations certainly suggest that they are well suited to serve as partners for health care organizations interested in improving the health of their communities, but an important question remains: How do clergy and members of religious institutions feel about devoting congregational time and resources to health programs?

To answer this question, we conducted two surveys (Hale and Bennett 2003). In both cases, we were surprised by the high level of interest. In our first study, we had the opportunity to survey clergy who were attending a weeklong continuing education program. This program drew clergy from more than twenty states and a dozen denominations. It is important to note that the focus of this program was not on health ministries or any health-related topic but on preaching and theology. We developed a questionnaire titled "Partnering with Hospitals: What Do You Think?" The pastors were asked to "assume that a hospital in your community wants to work with you to enhance the health of the members of your congregation. The hospital is offering various programs and services to you at no cost, but it does ask that you support its efforts by providing leadership and assistance in certain areas."

Ninety-eight pastors completed the survey. Three-fourths of these came from five denominations (Baptist, 20%; Lutheran, 17%; Methodist, 13%; Presbyterian, 13%; and Disciples of Christ, 11%). Seventy-two percent of the respondents said that it was "very important" for churches to actively address the health needs of their congregations. The remaining 28 percent said it was "somewhat important." None of the pastors felt that it was of little or no importance.

When we asked about specific health-related offerings, we found that 80 percent or more of these clergy favored using congregational facilities for screenings (e.g., blood pressure checks), preventive interventions (e.g., flu vaccinations), and health-related classes (e.g., nutrition, stress management). Eighty percent also said they would offer support for volunteers in their congregations trained to provide assistance for congregational members who needed help at home or when they visited their physician. Two-thirds of the clergy reported that they favored using congregational mailings or newsletters to announce the availability of screenings designed to detect serious medical conditions (e.g., hypertension, diabetes) and that they would personally encourage their congregation to participate in regular screenings.

We then surveyed more than five hundred members of religious congregations. Two-thirds of this group came from five religious groups: Baptist (19%), Methodist (17%), Presbyterian (12%), Catholic (11%), and Lutheran (10%). A brief paragraph at the top of their questionnaire stated, "Many hospitals and medical professionals would like to help churches (synagogues) address the health needs and concerns of their members. We would like to know if church (synagogue) members are interested in having health programs in their church (synagogue)."

Eighty-five percent reported that they would like to have educational programs on health matters presented at their church or synagogue, and 45 percent indicated they would be interested in helping organize or promote these health programs. The top choices for programs were:

Stress management, 56%
Alzheimer's disease (or other forms of dementia), 53%
Cancer, 51%
Heart disease, 48%
Depression, 48%
Cardiopulmonary resuscitation, 47%
Living wills, do not resuscitate orders, and other advance directives,
    45%
Arthritis, 40%

Diabetes, 38%
Healthy meal preparation, 37%
Hypertension, 35%
Stroke, 35%

When we asked about other types of health-related programs or concerns, we found that 78 percent wanted health screenings (e.g., blood pressure, blood sugar, cholesterol, or skin cancer) to be available at church, and 74 percent wanted preventive measures (e.g., flu vaccinations) to be offered. Eighty percent thought there were people in their congregation who needed more exercise and would be interested in joining a walking group or other exercise group that met regularly at their church (55 percent reported they would be interested in participating in such a program); 81 percent thought there were individuals in their church who may be depressed but were not getting the treatment or help they needed; and 82 percent thought there were individuals in their church who would benefit from being a member of a support group that meets regularly.

These surveys indicate strong support among clergy and laity for congregational health programs. Further evidence of the high level of support for congregational health programs among the religiously involved comes from a larger and more recent survey. The Baylor Religion Survey (2005), a nationally representative survey of 1,721 respondents that included nearly 400 items, provided an extensive and in-depth analysis of the religious beliefs and practices of Americans. One of the interesting findings of this study was that the most commonly held value among their respondents was taking care of the sick and needy. This ranked higher than teaching others your morals, converting others to your religious faith, or any of the other options. And this high level of support for taking care of the sick and needy cut across all religious and theological divisions.

PREVENTIVE MEDICINE

How can congregations merge their interest in health matters with the resources of health care organizations to produce effective health programs? Although health concerns will vary from congregation to congregation, we have found that the best way to begin planning for health programs is to adopt the basic principles and methods of *preventive medicine.*

This field is dedicated to preventing, or at least greatly reducing, the risk of premature illness, disability, and death. The key to effective preventive medicine programs is getting medical information and resources to people in a timely and easy-to-use fashion. The goal is to have everyone acquire a better understanding of what can be done to maintain health and ensure functional independence. In the remainder of this chapter, we review the basic concepts of preventive medicine and illustrate how these can be incorporated into the life and mission of religious congregations.

Preventive practices and interventions are generally organized into three categories or levels: primary, secondary, and tertiary. The following sections provide descriptions and examples of programs at each of these levels.

Primary Prevention

The goal of primary prevention is to prevent the development of disease and disability. By engaging in health-enhancing practices and avoiding health-compromising activities, people can greatly reduce their risk of developing various chronic diseases and experiencing serious injuries. Included in this category are both lifestyle modifications and immunizations. Some examples are giving up smoking, exercising regularly, eating properly, preventing injuries, and obtaining vaccinations against influenza, pneumonia, and tetanus.

One of the greatest challenges facing any organization sponsoring a primary prevention informational program is that many people do not pay attention to health matters until a serious illness or injury strikes. It is not easy to persuade people who are feeling healthy that they need to make lifestyle changes, especially when there are no immediate apparent benefits. Even when individuals believe that ignoring such advice may have negative consequences on their health, the current changes they need to make may seem too great or too costly because the likely harmful consequences of their behavior may not occur until much later in their lives.

Religious institutions have certain advantages when sponsoring primary prevention programs. First, they can incorporate information about primary prevention practices into regularly scheduled programs. In this way, they have a "built-in" audience. Second, they can present the information in different formats and at various times. This is important because one message alone is seldom sufficient to produce lasting changes in long-standing behavioral patterns. Most people need to hear such messages several times. Third, most religious congregations have members of all ages. This allows them to schedule intergenerational programs on health matters. They can encourage older adults, especially those who have chronic illnesses, to bring their children and even grandchildren to an informational program. Children and young adults are more likely to listen to and heed advice on illness prevention measures when they can see first-hand the impact of chronic diseases.

Examples of a Congregational Primary Prevention Program

A simple and yet effective primary prevention program you can sponsor for your congregation and community is one that encourages older adults to get annual influenza vaccinations. Even though in a typical year more than 35,000 deaths and 200,000 hospitalizations result from influenza and its complications (Centers for Disease Control and Prevention 2007a), the vaccination rate among adults 65 and older has remained flat at only about 60–70 percent for the last ten years, despite ongoing national efforts to increase the vaccination rate among this vulnerable group. Non-Hispanic whites continue to have higher vaccination rates than African Americans and other racial and ethnic groups (Centers for Disease Control and Prevention 2007b), reflecting a pattern of health disparity seen in other measures of preventive health care in the United States. In spite of the grave dangers associated with influenza and substantial evidence for the effectiveness of the vaccine, large numbers of older adults fail to get annual vaccinations. Education programs sponsored jointly by congregations and respected health organizations can increase the number of vaccinations and decrease the number of hospitalizations and deaths due to influenza. Participation can be increased even more by arranging for the health department or a hospital to offer vaccinations after the worship service or other well-attended congregational programs.

Another example of primary prevention is Westminster by-the-Sea Presbyterian Church's program designed to prevent falls, the number one cause of injuries and hospital admissions for trauma among older adults. By providing members with suggestions for making their homes safer, encouraging those whose medical condition places them at risk for falls to use assistive devices, and lending out walkers and wheelchairs, the program is able to provide services shown to reduce the risk of injuries, hospitalizations, early admission to nursing homes, and even death.

Secondary Prevention

The goal of secondary prevention is to detect a disease in its earliest stages in order to cure it or slow its progression. Screening tests can identify some medical conditions (e.g., diabetes) before symptoms become evident. Once a diagnosis is made, treatment can begin and the progression of the disease and its complications may be slowed or prevented. In this way the development of disability can be slowed and life can even be prolonged. Once a disease or condition has been detected, interventions may include strictly medical measures or some of the lifestyle modifications listed in the section on primary prevention. Recommended screenings generally include breast cancer, colorectal cancer, skin cancer, hypertension, hypercholesterolemia, diabetes, and depression and potential for suicide.

Time and transportation can be barriers to secondary prevention. Many people complain that they do not have the time in their busy schedules to participate in medical screenings and counseling, particularly when they are feeling healthy. Other individuals, especially many older adults, may have the time for screenings but find it difficult to arrange transportation. Religious congregations can help people overcome both of these barriers by arranging for screenings to be conducted on-site and in conjunction with regularly scheduled congregational gatherings. Hospitals, home health agencies, and physicians can be enlisted to assist in these screenings. If you cannot arrange to have screenings conducted in your congregational facilities, you can still facilitate the screenings by arranging for transportation to and from the local hospital or medical laboratory.

Examples of Congregational Secondary Prevention Programs

A simple, inexpensive secondary prevention program that can be sponsored by a religious congregation is one in which volunteer nurses or health care specialists provide blood pressure checks before or after the worship service. Little time and equipment are needed for this program, but it can yield meaningful results. By identifying people with high blood pressure and encouraging them to take appropriate measures to bring their blood pressure under control, you can reduce the incidence of heart attacks and strokes. Announcements in congregational bulletins and from respected congregational leaders can increase the number of people participating in and benefiting from this program.

Another example of a secondary prevention program is the skin cancer screening that is a regular event at Westminster by-the-Sea Presbyterian Church. The high level of participation in this valuable program is the result of reliable information about skin cancer, the strong endorsement of Rev. Sumner, and the fact that the screenings are conducted immediately after the Sunday worship service.

Tertiary Prevention

The goal of tertiary prevention is to reduce the complications and disabilities associated with existing disease. This is often referred to by health professionals as disease or illness *management*. Patients and their families need to learn how to manage chronic medical conditions effectively. Appropriate management can help patients live longer and maintain their independence and quality of life. Some preventive measures at the tertiary level are:

- Identifying and using appropriate medical services
- Complying with recommendations about medication
- Using community resources to enhance functional health
- Sponsoring support groups for patients and families

Religious congregations are ideal for numerous types of tertiary prevention programs. Many people who have chronic conditions fail to receive appropriate treatments and related services because they do not know about various community resources. Clergy and lay leaders are usually aware of community medical services and other community agencies, often serving in leadership roles in these organizations. They can compile and pass along the information to members who need these services. Also, to ensure that members who live alone are doing well, many congregations have programs in which volunteers regularly check up on them by telephone. These volunteers can also be easily trained to use these contacts to remind members about their medication. Support groups for patients or families also fit well within the mission and ministry of most congregations.

Examples of Congregational Tertiary Prevention Programs

One way a congregation can assist in tertiary prevention (or disease management) is to sponsor a support group for people with a specific condition or for their families experiencing disease-related stress. These groups can be helpful in many ways. Some people find it difficult to follow through with their treatment regimens on a consistent basis once the crisis seems to have passed. For example, some heart patients will revert to unhealthy dietary practices or abandon regular exercise programs once they feel they have recovered from a heart attack. Support groups can give these people and their families and caregivers the assistance and support they need to maintain their new regimens. Support groups can also help patients and their loved ones cope with some of the limitations and emotional aspects of an illness. Often new coping strategies can be learned from other members of the group.

The programs on medication management sponsored by Westminster by-the-Sea Presbyterian Church, particularly the ones addressing cholesterol-lowering medications, are another good example of a simple yet important approach to tertiary prevention. A common mistake made by individuals taking cholesterol-lowering medications is that, once their cholesterol levels have reached the desired range, they believe they do not need to continue taking the medication. Having pharmacists and physicians explain how these medications work and the need for people to continue taking them after their cholesterol levels have reached the target levels—unless their physicians instruct them to discontinue the medication—can reduce the risk of heart attack.

3

CONGREGATIONAL

HEALTH EDUCATION PROGRAMS

One of the most valuable and meaningful programs that can be offered to a congregation and community is a proactive health education program. Information is at the heart of both health promotion and illness management. People of all ages, even children, need to know more about health, illnesses, and medical care. Most of the life-limiting and life-threatening diseases encountered in middle or late adulthood have roots in earlier years. Members of your congregation and community need clear, reliable information about steps they can take to promote wellness and reduce the risks of developing illnesses. Congregants who already have medical conditions need reliable information about how they can effectively manage their conditions, reduce the likelihood of developing disability, and even prolong life.

LINKING PEOPLE AND INFORMATION

Physicians, psychologists, and other researchers in the field of preventive medicine have developed a large body of scientific information about the steps people can take to prevent illnesses or at least lessen their impact. There is reliable information about the activities or practices that increase the odds of staying healthy as well as those that increase the odds of developing chronic illnesses. There are also well-established methods for detecting many diseases in the early stages, thus limiting their harmful effects.

Most of this information about health promotion, early detection programs, and illness management is straightforward and easy for people to understand. You do not have to possess in-depth knowledge about the biological or medical aspects of most illnesses to understand what types of activity will enhance your health and what types may compromise your health. Nor do you have to understand exactly how medical examinations are analyzed to receive the benefits of regular monitoring of certain key measures of your health.

Although most of the information we need about health matters is easy to understand, too many of us fail to take advantage of it. Either we do not obtain the necessary information, or we fail to act on it. Why? The reasons vary from person to person, and we need to understand and be sensitive to these reasons as we plan and implement a health education program.

OVERCOMING BARRIERS TO WELLNESS PROMOTION

Some people simply are not motivated to seek out information on health matters until a medical crisis arises. As long as they feel well, they are not interested in reading materials or attending programs on health issues. These individuals either are not aware of or not concerned about the eventual consequences of their health-compromising actions. In fact, studies have found that although health is generally ranked at or near the top of values people hold, somewhere between 20 and 40 percent of people do not rank it in their top five (Ware and Young 1979).

Some individuals say they ignore information on health matters because they are confused by the various warnings and recommendations, which often seem contradictory, and they do not know what to believe. Others believe the information they have heard is reliable, but they are not motivated to act on it. They know that modifying some aspects of their lifestyle would be beneficial, but they cannot make the necessary changes. Sometimes they are too busy with other pressing responsibilities to focus on their health. Other people know what course of action they should take and make a decision to follow up on it, but then they have difficulty staying on track. This is not surprising because most of us find it hard to make lasting changes unless we receive regular reminders and ongoing encouragement and support.

Whatever the reasons, too many people fail to use valuable information on health to their advantage. In fact, one of the greatest challenges in health care is finding an effective means of delivering health information directly to the people who need it most, persuading them that they will benefit from this information, and providing the ongoing support they need to faithfully adhere to well-established prevention and treatment regimens. We must find innovative and appealing ways of reaching people.

Religious institutions, through their professional and lay leaders, can play a critical role in bringing information and people together. Congregational leaders have the ability to reach people *before* they encounter a medical crisis. Furthermore, they can present the information in ways that can be understood and appreciated by the members of their congregations and communities, and they can design informational programs that overcome many of the obstacles encountered in most community health education programs. These leaders have the potential to empower people by giving them the knowledge and tools to maintain their health and independence.

Although congregational leaders have many tangible and intangible resources that they can use in their efforts to minister to the health needs of their congregations, they still face significant challenges. Effective health education programs require a multifaceted, proactive approach. You have to do more than simply place attractive brochures in the pews.

First, you have to get people's attention. You have to find ways for the information you are providing to stand out from everything else people are reading and hearing. This is not always an easy task, but somehow you must reach out to them and convince them that you have information they need to hear. Second, you need to persuade them that there are decisions they can make and actions they can take that will yield personal health benefits. Third, you must convince them that the benefits of their decisions and actions outweigh the costs. Fourth, you need to bring them together in support of each other as they work to adopt and maintain health-enhancing actions.

THE HEALTH BELIEF MODEL

The most helpful model to use in planning is the health belief model (Rosenstock 1974). This simple model, widely used throughout the health care field, can help you organize the presentation of information such that it will have the greatest impact on your audiences. The four components of this model are presented below, followed by an example that applies the health belief model to hypertension.

First, you must convince people that they are susceptible to a disease or condition. People who are unaware that they are vulnerable to a particular disease (e.g., diabetes, hypertension, glaucoma) are not likely to take the correct steps to prevent its onset or detect it in the earliest stages.

Second, you need to persuade people that the disease or condition can have severe consequences. It is not enough for people to believe that they are susceptible to an illness; they must also realize that it can be seriously harmful. They must see that a particular disease or condition could greatly limit their ability to enjoy their favorite activities or even shorten their life. People who believe that they may be susceptible to a particular illness but do not believe that the illness can have severe consequences are unlikely to make any significant modifications in their lifestyle or health practices.

Third, people must believe in the efficacy or power of the prevention or treatment recommendations. You need to convince people that there are steps they can take to reduce the risk of becoming ill or to minimize the impact of a disease. If people believe that there are no effective treatments for a disease, they will see no reason to participate in early detection programs.

Fourth, people must believe that the benefits of illness prevention and treatment regimens outweigh the costs or burdens of those regimens. This point is often overlooked by health workers, who may not be aware of the perceived costs or burdens associated with certain actions. Although the benefits may seem obvious to health care professionals, many people feel that the costs associated with various treatments outweigh the benefits. Even small costs may be the primary reason that elderly or low-income persons do not seek services. This is where the feedback you receive from members of your congregation and community can be helpful in identifying barriers and then finding ways to overcome them. Working together, health care organizations and religious congregations may be able to find creative ways to reduce the costs or burdens associated with certain services.

One additional variable thought to be important is an instigating event or cue to action. This could be a public awareness campaign or the testimony of a person who benefited by taking the recommended action (e.g., receiving treatment for a medical condition detected through a health screening).

Health education programs that are designed with these objectives in mind are most likely to have an impact on members of your congregation and community.

Hypertension, or high blood pressure, can illustrate how the health belief model can be used to organize educational programs. Many people are unaware of the problem of high blood pressure or do not know they are susceptible to it. Some people believe they are in good health—free of any disease—as long as they do not have any painful symptoms. They do not think they need to concern themselves with getting their blood pressure checked unless they begin to feel ill. Therefore, the first step in educating and helping them change their health practices is to find some way to convince them that they are susceptible to hypertension, even if they are not feeling ill or experiencing high levels of stress.

One way to help people understand that they are susceptible to hypertension is to give them information about its widespread prevalence. Once they realize that millions of people have hypertension but are unaware of their condition, they may be more willing to acknowledge the possibility that they too could have high blood pressure. This type of information may also help catch the attention of specific groups of people who are known to have high rates of hypertension, such as African Americans. Another way to reach and influence people is to share examples of people similar to them who discovered they had high blood pressure. Often a few such personal examples are more effective than statistics. When possible, it is best to use a combination of these two approaches because some people respond best to statistical information, while others respond best to personal accounts.

Second, you need to persuade people that there are potentially severe consequences associated with hypertension. Individuals who are aware of the problem of hypertension but believe that there are no serious effects associated with it are not likely to monitor their blood pressure regularly and seek treatment should it be too high. They may view it as a condition that has little significance for their overall health. Other people may attempt to dismiss the risks associated with hypertension by saying, "I have to die of something." Often this is a way of avoiding a threatening subject, but such a statement also indicates that they are overlooking serious consequences other than death. These people need to be reminded that high blood pressure increases their risk of heart attack and stroke, both of which may leave them seriously disabled. Although they may survive, they may be left in a condition in which they are unable to participate in many of the activities they enjoy and find rewarding. The prospect of a long-term disability is often viewed as a more undesirable outcome than death.

Third, once you have made people understand that they are susceptible to hypertension and that it can have severe consequences, you need to persuade them that there are things they can do to help themselves. You need to offer hope and educate people about the steps to take to reduce the risk of hypertension and its potentially harmful consequences. They need to hear from reliable, authoritative sources that by making certain lifestyle modifications or taking medication, they can bring their blood pressure under control.

Fourth, you must be sensitive to people's perceptions about the cost of following the recommended prevention, monitoring, and treatment regimens for hypertension. Some people may believe the financial costs of treatment outweigh the benefits, especially if they are on a limited budget and have other financial obligations. Others may fear that the side effects of the medication for their blood pressure will actually produce a poorer quality of life. Sometimes fears about the costs or negative effects of treatment are based on erroneous beliefs that can be corrected by providing accurate information from an authoritative source. However, in some situations, costs can be a real factor. In such cases, you may be able to give information about professionals or agencies that can provide less costly treatments or offer financial assistance.

The cues to action for a congregational program on hypertension could begin with a bulletin insert with basic information on hypertension—its prevalence, the potentially harmful consequences if not treated, and treatment options. This could be supplemented by a brief presentation by a member of the congregation who discovered through a health screening that in spite of feeling healthy he or she had hypertension. Finally, blood pressure checks could be provided immediately before or after the congregational gathering.

MOTIVATING PEOPLE TO MAKE CHANGES

The health belief model can be useful in designing programs and materials for your congregation. It should help as you select topics and decide what type of information needs to be presented to your congregation or community. However, although many members of your congregation will appreciate your work, your efforts may not be warmly received or appreciated by all. You may encounter resistance or criticism from others in the congregation. Some individuals may feel that you are being critical or judgmental when you encourage them to make changes in their lifestyle. Often people who have the greatest need to adopt new practices are the most difficult to reach. It takes a sensitive and diplomatic approach in the presentation of information to overcome this resistance. Even those who are aware that they need to alter their lifestyle or behavioral patterns are often ambivalent about change. They may genuinely want to be healthy and know that they would benefit from the recommended changes, but they also realize that by making these changes they would be giving up certain activities or habits that they enjoy. Therefore, it is a good idea to know some basic principles and strategies that can be applied when you are encouraging people to adopt new health practices and to abandon, or at least modify, some longstanding habits.

Two books on motivational interviewing—*Motivational Interviewing: Preparing People for Change,* by Miller and Rollnick, and *Motivational Interviewing in Health Care,* by Rollnick, Miller, and Butler—provide a good model appropriate for work in congregations. Although the principles and strategies they offer are generally used by health professionals working on a one-to-one basis, they are also appropriate for working with groups of people who need encouragement as they seek to incorporate health-enhancing practices into their lifestyle and discard or reduce health-compromising habits.

The first principle of motivational interviewing is to *express empathy.* People are more open to change when they sense that you have a good understanding of their situation and the stresses and challenges they face in their life. They are more likely to listen to you and accept the information you are offering if they can tell that you understand how they feel. The steps you or your speakers recommend may seem both obvious and simple to you but may strike some people as overwhelming, at least given their current circumstances. To be truly empathic, it is necessary to listen carefully and with an open mind when these individuals express their feelings and concerns about what is being recommended. You need to be willing to put yourself in their position and be able to view life from their perspective. This does not mean that you must agree with everything they say, but it does mean that you need to convey to them that you accept their actions, thoughts, and feelings without judging them or criticizing them.

The second principle is to *develop discrepancy.* Although listening carefully and empathizing with people is an important and usually necessary first step in helping them to change, it is often not sufficient. For people to become motivated to actually make changes, they need to recognize that there is a discrepancy between where they are now with respect to health-enhancing practices and where they could be. They need to understand that they will fail to achieve some worthwhile goals if they continue their current practices. The awareness of this discrepancy is what can provide the fuel or energy for change. But it is important that this perceived discrepancy be between their current state and *their* goals, not yours. They need to see the connection between the things in life they care about and their health behaviors. Therefore, you can be helpful by aiding them in identifying some goals that they truly value. These goals can vary tremendously. For some individuals, the goal of being able to live longer than their parents or with fewer health-related limitations may be best, whereas for others the goal of being able to enjoy activities with their grandchildren may be the most important.

The third principle is to *avoid argumentation.* When people feel they are being directly attacked or criticized for "bad habits" or "problem behaviors," they are likely to become defensive and develop arguments that they believe justify their current practices. Even arguing that someone *should* have a particular goal or *should* follow certain practices can lead to resistance. Instead, keep the emphasis on the positive—the benefits of adopting some of the recommendations about how to become healthier. The objective of a good health education program is not to make people feel bad about their current health status but to inspire people to become healthier. You want to help people find their own reasons and rewards for avoiding health-compromising activities and adopting health-enhancing practices.

The fourth principle is to *roll with resistance.* Do not be surprised when people seem to ignore the information and services you are offering them. Not everyone is going to appreciate what you are trying to accomplish. But do not give up. Be flexible. Approach the topic from a different perspective, or focus on another topic. If people object to your approach or seem uninterested, ask them what type of information they want or what format for health education programs is the most appealing. Listen to their feedback and involve them in your planning process. In most situations, your audience can give you helpful advice about how to approach them.

The fifth principle is to *support self-efficacy.* People need to develop the belief that they have the capacity, the power, to make changes. It is important for them to see that they can be successful in making constructive modifications in their life. Successful experiences, even small successes, can help people build this sense of self-efficacy. Therefore, it is helpful to encourage people to set reasonable goals for themselves. People with sedentary lifestyles do not have to join the local gym and become great athletes; they simply need to increase their physical activities. Any increase should be viewed as a success. Similarly, people who have become accustomed to a diet high in fat do not have to adopt a strict low-fat diet to be successful; they need only to reduce some of the fat in their diet to rightfully claim success. Movement in the right direction, even if it comes in small steps, can build confidence and raise expectations about their ability to make additional changes.

ON-SITE SERVICES AND SUPPORTIVE FOLLOW-UP

When planning health programs for your congregation or community, recognize the value of on-site services. Some of the steps you or your guest speakers are recommending may seem too costly financially or in terms of time if people have to leave work or make special travel arrangements. For example, some individuals may be persuaded that it would be wise to monitor their blood pressure on a regular basis, but they find it difficult to get to their doctor's office or a clinic. Problems with transportation or scheduling may prevent them from regular visits. An easy solution to these problems is to arrange for nurses to provide blood pressure checks once every month or two immediately after a worship service or a regularly scheduled congregational meeting. Providing on-site services will lessen the cost or burden of following the health-enhancing recommendations people have received in your educational programs. Anything you can do to remove or reduce barriers will increase the chances of people engaging in health-enhancing activities.

Finally, the value of regular reminders and supportive follow-up services cannot be emphasized enough. People are not always ready for the information you are offering at the time you are offering it. For example, many individuals may not think they need to know much about depression the first time you provide information on mood disorders in a congregational program because it does not seem to be a factor in their life or the lives of their loved ones. However, a few months later they may be ready to hear about the topic because a family member or friend is showing signs of depression. Another reason to incorporate regular messages and reminders is that most people find it difficult to make lasting changes in their behavior patterns and health practices. Friendly reminders can help them stay on track and maintain their motivation.

II

SUGGESTED TOPICS FOR
CONGREGATIONAL PROGRAMS

4

CORONARY HEART DISEASE

Coronary heart disease is the leading cause of death in the United States. Each year approximately 1.5 million Americans suffer a heart attack and nearly half a million die as a result of the attack. Heart attacks (myocardial infarctions) occur when arterial (blood vessel) blockages stop blood and oxygen from reaching the heart muscle—as when a clogged fuel line stops a car engine. The blockage is generally due to atherosclerosis, or the build-up of plaque in the arteries. The process of plaque building up and causing a thickening and narrowing of the arteries begins long before a heart attack occurs. In fact, it is a gradual process that may start as early as childhood. It is increasingly recognized that some heart attacks occur due to rupture of atherosclerotic plaques—even those that before rupturing do not obstruct the flow of blood through the affected artery. When a plaque ruptures, the rapid formation of a clot occurs and the artery can become completely blocked. Whatever the underlying physiology, rapid medical treatment in a hospital with "clot-busting" drugs and angioplasty (where a balloon catheter can be used to open the clogged coronary artery) not only saves lives but also lessens the heart muscle damage that follows the event.

RISK FACTORS FOR CORONARY HEART DISEASE

The major risk factors for coronary artery disease are age, sex, family history, high cholesterol, hypertension, diabetes mellitus, and smoking. Heart disease is more common among older adults. In fact, of all the known risk factors for heart disease, older age is the most potent. Not only does plaque form more readily in older arteries, but the arteries of older adults have been exposed to the other important risk factors (e.g., hypertension, high cholesterol, and smoking) for a longer period of time. Finally, the incidence rates of hypertension and diabetes, two common late-life conditions among people in the United States, increase dramatically among older age groups and may further accelerate the worsening of coronary artery disease. In addition, older adults are also more vulnerable to heart disease and regularly have more complications and worse outcomes as compared to younger patients. For these reasons, knowledge of the risk and early recognition and treatment of heart disease are especially important among older people.

Heart disease is more common in men than in women during early and middle adulthood, but the risk of heart disease rises dramatically in postmenopausal women after the age of 50. Although many women fear breast cancer as the number one cause of death, heart disease affects and kills many more women than all forms of cancer combined. For both women and men, heredity also plays an important role because the risk of heart disease is greater for those with a family history of premature heart attacks. For individuals who do not know their family history, efforts at establishing such a family health record is recommended. High levels of blood cholesterol can also run in families, and many medical studies now support the identification and treatment of high cholesterol as an effective strategy in the prevention and treatment of coronary artery disease.

One of the most common risks for heart disease, particularly in older adults, is hypertension, or high blood pressure. As we age, our arteries naturally get stiffer. Thus, hypertension often develops after 50 years of age, even among those with good exercise and nutritional habits. Women develop hypertension with aging but about a decade later than men. Up to 70 percent of 70-year-olds and 80 percent of 80-year-olds have high blood pressure. The type of hypertension that develops in older age is different from hypertension that is diagnosed at younger ages; it is far more risky. Treatment of hypertension associated with the aging process markedly reduces the risk of stroke, heart attack, death, heart failure, kidney disease, and even dementia. Therefore, it is important to have blood pressure checked on a regular basis to avoid or lessen the risk of developing these conditions. People also become more sensitive to salt in older age. Because salt increases blood pressure, learning to lower the salt in one's diet by cooking and choosing food products with less salt can also help to lower blood pressure.

Developing diabetes is a potent predictor of future heart disease. Because obesity is a significant risk factor for diabetes (and hypertension), being overweight is an important risk factor for coronary artery disease as well. Physicians recognize the "metabolic syndrome" as a combination of obesity, high blood pressure, and abnormally high blood glucose or diabetes. One of the simplest predictors of this syndrome's development is the measurement of waist size. Waist sizes greater than 40 inches for men and greater than 35 inches for women are highly predictive of development of metabolic syndrome and the ultimate development of adverse health outcomes. (See www.cdc.gov/nchs/data/nhanes/bm.pdf for instruction in measuring waist size.) Programs that address maintenance of a healthy weight and identify and control blood glucose levels and diabetes are particularly important for preventing and treating coronary artery disease.

Finally, besides its deleterious effects on lung function and recognized role in causing multiple cancer types, smoking is a very significant risk factor for heart disease, and stopping smoking is clearly the most potent *modifiable* risk-reduction strategy for delaying the development of coronary artery disease.

THE RISKS OF IGNORING INFORMATION ON HEART DISEASE

The most serious and feared consequence of failing to heed information about heart disease is a fatal heart attack. Each year approximately half a million persons die as a result of a heart attack, many of them older adults. However, many people fail to realize that there may be grave and long-lasting consequences for those who survive a heart attack. Heart failure, most commonly caused by damaged heart muscle following a heart attack, is a serious condition and the leading cause of hospitalization among older adults. In this condition, the heart muscle is too weak to pump enough blood forward to provide the body with the oxygen it needs to meet the demands of normal activities. In addition, when blood cannot be pumped forward efficiently, it often "backs up" into the lungs, causing severe shortness of breath. The lives of people with heart failure are usually seriously limited due to the fatigue, weakness, and shortness of breath associated with this condition. For the most affected individuals, even limited physical exertion like walking around one's bedroom can produce shortness of breath.

WHAT CAN BE DONE TO PREVENT HEART DISEASE?
Reducing the Risk

Many steps can be taken to avoid, or at least greatly delay, the harmful consequences of heart disease. The most important ones that are within one's control include changes in lifestyle:

- *Stop smoking.* Smoking contributes to heart disease by promoting the build-up of plaque in the arteries. It is not easy for most people to stop smoking, but the benefits are significant. Even after a lifetime of smoking, quitting at any age greatly reduces the risk of future heart disease.
- *Decrease the amount of cholesterol and saturated fat in your diet.* Knowing the different types of fat and avoiding or limiting the foods that are high in saturated fat is the first place to start. Information can be obtained on package labels. If dietary changes are not sufficient to lower cholesterol to acceptable levels, several effective medications can be taken.
- *Exercise more often.* You do not have to embark on a rigorous and exhausting exercise program, but it does need to be regular. Walking for 20 to 30 minutes a day is optimal. Try to walk places instead of riding when possible.
- *Lose weight.* If you are overweight, lose weight by participating in a safe, gradual weight reduction program. Fad diets usually do not work in the long run.
- *Have regular check-ups.* Many of the conditions that lead to heart disease develop in the later years. These include hypertension and diabetes. Often these conditions develop without any signs or symptoms, so it is important to get your blood pressure and blood sugar checked regularly, either by your doctor or at health fairs. By making regular visits to the doctor, you may also be able to avoid a

stroke because flow obstruction in your carotid arteries (located on either side on the front of your neck) can sometimes be heard by your physician. Regular testing of cholesterol is also important, particularly for younger adults with other risk factors for heart disease, and for everyone diagnosed with coronary artery disease. Your physician might also recommend taking an aspirin tablet daily, depending on your overall risk profile for heart disease.

Detecting the Early Signs of Coronary Heart Disease

Detecting coronary heart disease can be difficult because the atherosclerotic process can be well advanced before there are any noticeable signs of heart disease. For example, the pain and discomfort associated with myocardial ischemia (an inadequate flow of blood to part of the heart) may not occur until the artery is narrowed by 75 percent. This chest pain or discomfort is referred to as angina pectoris and occurs when there is ischemia in that the demand for blood and oxygen by the heart muscle exceeds the supply delivered by the narrowed artery. Angina usually occurs during activity and goes away with rest. Older persons sometimes do not experience chest discomfort with ischemia. Instead, they can have shortness of breath during activity that resolves shortly after resting. Other ways in which anginal symptoms may present in older patients are activity-related neck, arm, or throat pain or burning; nausea; cold sweats; and/or dizziness.

Recognizing and Reacting to Signs of a Heart Attack

Thus far, we have discussed what can be done to reduce the risk of a heart attack. But what should be done if someone is having a heart attack? What are the symptoms? How quickly should you react and whom should you call if you think it is a heart attack?

The steps taken during the first minutes of a suspected heart attack are extremely important. They can make the difference between life and death or long-term disability. Immediate emergency medical attention is necessary. Therefore, it is important for people to know the early signs of a heart attack. These are the warning signals:

- Chest pain—frequently described as pressure or squeezing sensations
- Pain spreading to shoulders, arms (especially the left arm), and jaw
- Sudden feeling of faintness or breathlessness
- Nausea and vomiting
- Sweating

Often older adults do not have significant chest discomfort during a heart attack and may simply have shortness of breath, confusion, dizziness, nausea, and cold sweats.

If these warning signs are experienced for more than a few minutes emergency medical care should be sought immediately. Call 911 and do not drive or have someone drive you to the hospital. Recent research supports that taking one aspirin tablet—as long as one is not allergic to aspirin—might slow the clot formation that causes heart attacks.

SUGGESTIONS FOR CONGREGATIONAL PROGRAMS

Provide assistance for members of your congregation and community who want to stop smoking. This assistance can be in the form of information on smoking cessation programs available in your community or classes offered at one of your congregation's facilities. Your hospital and the American Heart Association can give you information about programs and materials.

Provide information on nutrition and offer samples of low-fat meals and snacks. There are several ways to do this:

1. Have a special program on this topic, with a dietitian offering information on food selection and meal preparation.
2. Incorporate low-fat foods into regularly scheduled congregational meals and then distribute information about the low-fat food items to those in attendance.
3. Arrange for a dietitian to offer a series of cooking classes in which the emphasis is on the preparation of low-fat, low-salt, heart-healthy meals.
4. Have a group in the congregation prepare a book of recipes on heart-healthy meals.

In all of these approaches, demonstrate that it is possible to have appealing, tasty meals that are also beneficial to one's health. The American Heart Association and a dietitian from the hospital can serve as valuable resources for these programs.

Sponsor a special program on heart disease. If possible, have a physician as your guest speaker. Although a cardiologist may seem like an obvious choice, family practitioners and internists are well prepared to speak on the subject of heart disease. This is also a good opportunity to offer blood pressure screenings and samples of low-fat, low-salt foods. Often grocery stores will donate food for these programs.

Provide assistance for people who want to participate in a program of regularly scheduled physical activity. This can be done by distributing information on exercise programs available in your community or by sponsoring a program held in one of your congregation's facilities. Something as simple as a walking club or group that meets regularly can prove beneficial and even fun for members who wish to incorporate physical activity into their schedule. The American Heart Association can provide materials for individuals who wish to design their own exercise programs.

Offer a workshop or class on stress management. Your hospital or a local mental health professional should be able to assist you in developing this program. Yoga classes are another method for practicing stress reduction as well as providing physical activity.

Offer a cardiopulmonary resuscitation (CPR) class for members of your congregation. The American Heart Association or your local hospital can help arrange for CPR training. Encourage older adults and those who live with older adults to attend this class.

Arrange for a class on automated external defibrillators (AEDs) to be offered to members of your congregation. The class could include instruction on where to look for AEDs (e.g., airports, shopping malls, sports arenas, etc.) and how to operate them.

Purchase one or more AEDs for your congregational facilities and arrange for several volunteers to receive training in how to operate them. The American Heart Association provides AED training through its network of Training Centers. Your local hospital also may be able to assist with the training.

Distribute cards describing the symptoms of a heart attack and instructions about how to respond to these symptoms. These cards can be obtained from the American Heart Association.

Arrange for the congregation to offer a heart health fair with blood pressure and cholesterol screening, heart disease information, and nutrition booths. The American Heart Association or your local hospital has resources to conduct these fairs.

Form a support group for those with heart disease and their family members. This can be helpful to form exercise groups, exchange nutritional tips, and reduce stress.

Use congregational bulletins and mailings to provide members of your congregation with basic information on heart disease and regular reminders to have their blood pressure and cholesterol levels checked. Your local chapter of the American Heart Association should be able to provide you with copies of brochures and booklets for distribution to your members.

EXAMPLES OF CONGREGATIONAL PROGRAMS

A special program on heart disease was held on a Saturday morning at St. Peter Catholic Church in DeLand, Florida. Dr. Frank Reed, a cardiologist and member of the church, was the featured speaker for the program. Before Dr. Reed spoke, those in attendance had an opportunity to have their blood pressure checked and to sample some low-fat snacks. The priest opened the program, offering a prayer and encouraging the audience to heed the doctor's advice. Dr. Reed then spoke, using a slide show prepared by the American Heart Association to illustrate his talk. This was followed by a question-and-answer period, a brief break during which people could talk to the doctor on a one-to-one basis, and finally a short presentation on nutrition by a speaker from the American Heart Association. Most people stayed for the entire program, and many commented on how helpful it had been.

Of course, it is not always possible to coordinate your congregation's schedule with that of physicians or other professionals. One potential solution to scheduling difficulties is the use of video presentations. Dr. Donald Stoner, a cardiologist in Daytona Beach, strongly believed in the value of congregational health education programs and wished to assist as much as possible. However, he knew that he would not be able to accept all the invitations he received from congregations participating in the lay health education program sponsored by Halifax Health Medical Center, the hospital where he serves as chief medical officer. To overcome this problem, he prepared a video in which he spoke on hypertension and heart disease. This video proved to be a popular and valuable part of the health education program.

Mt. Bethel Baptist Institutional Church, an African American congregation in Daytona Beach, wanted to include a presentation on heart disease and hypertension during a regularly scheduled church program. When Dr. Stoner was unable to attend this program, they simply brought his message to the audience of 25 by showing his video. His message was reinforced by the volunteer lay health educator who coordinated the program and the pastor, who encouraged members to follow Dr. Stoner's advice. Several members of the audience responded positively to the talk, including one woman who gave a personal example of the dangers of not recognizing the symptoms of a heart attack. She related how her father died a few hours after complaining of indigestion, having failed to recognize that he was having a heart attack and needed emergency medical care. She also mentioned that Dr. Stoner's presentation had convinced her that she needed to resume the exercise program she had started shortly after her father's death.

INFORMATION RESOURCES

You can obtain many of the materials you will need for your programs on heart disease by contacting the local chapter of the American Heart Association. You can locate the nearest chapter of the American Heart Association by calling 1-800-AHA-USA-1 (1-800-242-8721) or visiting the organization's Web site (www.americanheart.org), where you will also find helpful information and additional materials. The American Heart Association or your local hospital can also help you identify professionals, volunteers, and other organizations in your community that offer services such as training in CPR, blood pressure checks, smoking cessation classes and support groups, cholesterol level testing, and guest speakers.

During the month of February, the American Heart Association sponsors a national campaign to raise the public's awareness of heart disease. You may wish to schedule some of your programs to coincide with this national educational effort.

Additional information on heart disease can be found at the following Internet Web sites:

www.nhlbi.nih.gov (National Heart, Lung, and Blood Institute)
www.cdc.gov/heartdisease (Centers for Disease Control and
    Prevention)

5

HYPERTENSION

Hypertension, or high blood pressure, is generally defined as a systolic pressure of 140 mm Hg or higher or a diastolic pressure of 90 mm Hg or higher. In more recent years, "prehypertension" has been recognized as a diagnosis among adults with systolic blood pressures in the 120–139 range, and diastolic blood pressures in the 80–89 range. Prehypertension often precedes the development of hypertension, but even at these lower levels, blood pressure accelerates damage in the normally elastic arteries. Also, by increasing the work of the heart pumping against high blood pressure, hypertension can ultimately lead to heart failure—even in the absence of atherosclerosis.

Hypertension affects approximately 50 million Americans, but only about half know they have this condition. The prevalence of hypertension increases with age. It is estimated that approximately 60 percent of Americans aged 60 or older have hypertension. Hypertension is more common among men than women before age 55, is roughly equivalent for men and women during the next two decades, but becomes a greater risk for women after age 74. It is most common in African Americans. Obese individuals and those with a family history of hypertension also are more likely to be affected by hypertension.

THE RISKS OF IGNORING INFORMATION
ON HYPERTENSION

Although hypertension frequently produces no symptoms, it can have many harmful consequences, including severe disability and death. Hypertension damages large and small arteries directly. This damage leads to disease in the tissues and organs receiving blood from the arteries. People with hypertension are at risk for stroke, heart disease, and kidney failure leading to dialysis. Longstanding hypertension can initially cause the heart to hypertrophy (or become overdeveloped and thickened), resulting in reduced pumping action, and eventually to dilate and weaken. This condition is called heart failure. People with heart failure tire easily and experience shortness of breath with minor exertion.

WHAT CAN BE DONE TO PREVENT HYPERTENSION AND ITS COMPLICATIONS?

The development of high blood pressure can likely be delayed through a number of lifestyle modifications including weight loss, regular exercise (both aerobic and low intensity), consumption of a diet low in salt and animal fat and rich in vegetables and fruit, and lowered alcohol intake. Studies have not shown that stress reduction programs or use of dietary nutritional supplements (e.g., fish oil, magnesium, fiber) can effectively prevent development of hypertension. Because high blood pressure is an independent risk factor for the development of cardiovascular disease, prevention programs should also address other lifestyle modifications, including smoking cessation and control of hypercholesterolemia.

Hypertension often goes undetected because it may produce no symptoms until it seriously damages the heart, brain, or kidneys. Some people with hypertension report headaches, but generally hypertension is discovered during routine checks or medical examinations. Fortunately, the assessment of blood pressure is easy and inexpensive. The major challenge health professionals face is persuading people that they should have their blood pressure checked on a regular basis and that they should seek treatment if they are found to have hypertension. Given the increasing numbers of young adults and children with obesity, assessment of blood pressure should be done even for younger individuals on a regular basis.

The good news about hypertension is that the interventions that can be used to prevent it also treat it. Once diagnosed, lifestyle modifications are frequently effective in controlling blood pressure. These include weight loss, restriction of salt intake, and exercise. Reduced alcohol consumption and potassium supplementation may also be useful interventions. Lifestyle modifications are generally recommended as an initial method of controlling blood pressure, but if such modifications are insufficient to bring blood pressure under control, numerous medications are available. Often more than one medication is required, and achieving successful control can take a number of weeks or months and multiple visits to your doctor.

Poor compliance with recommended interventions is a significant problem in the treatment of hypertension. Studies have shown that as many as half of patients who begin treatment for hypertension fail to continue. There are many reasons for this problem. Because many people do not have any symptoms associated with their high blood pressure and because the benefits of blood pressure control accrue over many years, an individual may have little tangible daily motivation to continue with the lifestyle changes or medication. Regular education about the benefits of maintaining healthier living patterns and being compliant with medications acts as reinforcement to improve compliance among such people. In addition, some people taking blood pressure medications report they feel better when they are not taking these drugs, and changes in therapy should be pursued for such individuals. If the cost of the medications prescribed is a deterrent to compliance, effective and less costly generic antihypertensives are typically available and can be substituted for the more expensive drugs. Thus, given the opportunities for improving compliance, educational programs have much to offer.

SUGGESTIONS FOR CONGREGATIONAL PROGRAMS

Offer periodic blood pressure checks immediately before or after worship services or other congregational meetings. Active or retired nurses from your congregation should be able to provide this service. If not, hospitals and home health agencies usually can send a staff member to conduct these checks.

Give information about locations in the community where members can have their blood pressure checked. Drugstores as well as fire stations often offer free blood pressure checks on a regular basis.

Sponsor a special program on hypertension with a physician or nurse educator as your featured speaker. Materials for this program can be obtained from the American Heart Association.

Sponsor a special program on antihypertensive medications with a phar-

macist as your featured speaker. Encourage people to ask about their concerns. Ask the pharmacist to discuss less expensive drugs for treating hypertension and to address the economic burden of complying with prescribed regimens.

Use congregational bulletins and mailings to provide members with basic information on hypertension. This information can be obtained from the American Heart Association. Your local chapter should be able to provide you with copies of brochures and booklets for distribution to your members.

Use congregational bulletins and mailings to provide members with regular reminders about monitoring their blood pressure and complying with treatment recommendations.

Encourage people interested in controlling hypertension to participate in exercise and nutrition programs. Several suggestions for such programs are covered in chapter 4. A program on nutrition and hypertension could feature information on sodium. One of the topics covered could be advice on how to interpret the information on sodium provided on the labels of packaged food.

EXAMPLES OF CONGREGATIONAL PROGRAMS

A well-attended and successful program on hypertension was held at Mt. Carmel Missionary Baptist Church, in Daytona Beach, Florida. Volunteers from several nearby churches helped to organize and sponsor this program. These volunteers felt that many people in their congregations were unaware of how prevalent hypertension is among African Americans and how dangerous it is for hypertension to go untreated. The volunteers invited Dr. Stoner, a cardiologist and chief medical officer at Halifax Health Medical Center, the hospital where most members of the congregations received their medical care, to be the guest speaker at the Friday evening program. They also arranged to have volunteer nurses available to conduct blood pressure checks and distribute materials provided by the American Heart Association.

Dr. Stoner, the son of a Baptist minister, opened his presentation with an enthusiastic endorsement of the role churches can play in the health of their members and then described the basic nature of hypertension, explained why it increases the risk of heart attack and stroke, and offered information about the treatments available. The audience responded well to his presentation. A number of questions were asked, and several in the audience commented that they were definitely going to encourage family members and friends to get their blood pressure checked and to seek treatment if they were found to have hypertension. Following Dr. Stoner's presentation, the audience was invited to sample some of the heart-healthy snacks that the volunteers had prepared.

Bonnie Bullock, the parish nurse at Coronado Community Methodist Church, in New Smyrna Beach, Florida, and coordinator of the Parish Nurse Program sponsored by Bert Fish Medical Center, has made a special effort to inform her fellow parishioners of the dangers of hypertension and to offer monthly blood pressure checks immediately following each of the three Sunday worship services. When she realized that many in the congregation assumed they did not need to be concerned about their blood pressure as long as it was below 140/90, she began educating the congregation about the importance of detecting prehypertension (a systolic blood pressure of 120–139 or a diastolic blood pressure of 80–89) and taking measures to prevent it from developing into hypertension. She has written articles on this and many other health topics for the church's monthly newsletter. The articles are also printed separately and placed in the church's welcome center. Reminders to pick up these articles are placed in the church bulletin, and during the worship services the pastor makes a point to encourage members to read the articles and to take advantage of the monthly blood pressure checks.

INFORMATION RESOURCES

Your local chapter of the American Heart Association can provide many of the materials you will need for your programs. You can locate the nearest chapter of the American Heart Association by calling 1-800-AHA-USA-1 (1-800-242-8721) or visiting the organization's Web site (www .americanheart.org). The American Heart Association or your local hospital can also help you identify professionals, volunteers, and other organizations in your community that offer services such as blood pressure checks, smoking cessation classes and support groups, stroke rehabilitation classes, and guest speakers.

The following Web sites have information that may be useful in your programs:

www.stroke.org (National Stroke Association)
www.nhlbi.nih.gov (National Heart, Lung, and Blood Institute)
www.cdc.gov/bloodpressure (Centers for Disease Control and
    Prevention)

6

CANCER

There are more than one hundred types of cancer, all characterized by the uncontrolled growth and spread of abnormal cells. The most common types that can lead to death are prostate, breast, lung, and colon cancer, each of which typically begins as a discrete localized tumor (or mass) in the affected organ. Skin cancers are also common, particularly among older patients, but less frequently lead to death if identified and treated early. Some less common cancers of the bloodstream, such as lymphoma or leukemia, involve the body more generally at the time of presentation. Initially, most organ and skin cancers are localized, with cancer cells confined to their original site. Later, cancer cells may spread or metastasize to other sites. Treatment is more successful when cancer is localized; once cancer cells have spread, treatment is more difficult and less effective.

More than 1,400,000 new cases of cancer are diagnosed and approximately 550,000 deaths from cancer occur each year in the United States, making it the second leading cause of death in our country. The incidence and mortality rates for cancer are generally higher for African Americans than for non-Hispanic whites, reflecting differences in genetics, environmental exposure related to socioeconomic status, and ongoing health care disparity. Paralleling these differences, the five-year survival rate for cancer in African Americans is significantly lower than for non-Hispanic whites, due in large part to diagnosis occurring later in the disease process.

THE RISKS OF IGNORING INFORMATION ON CANCER

Fear and fatalism often interfere with people's obtaining accurate information about cancer and the appropriate tests and treatment options. Many individuals are so fearful of cancer that they do not want to know much about it or participate in screenings that might detect it. Often their fear is combined with a fatalistic view of cancer: they believe that there is little they can do to prevent it and that there are virtually no effective treatments. People need help in overcoming their fear and sense of hopelessness about cancer. In recent years, screening for cancer has become more precise, and early detection has reduced some cancer death rates. People need to know not only that there are steps they can take to reduce their risk of developing cancer but also that other steps can result in early detection and cure.

WHAT CAN BE DONE TO PREVENT CANCER?

It is important that cancer be detected and treated as early as possible. Generally, the earlier the treatment begins, the better the chance of curing or controlling the cancer. The overall survival rate for many cancers would increase significantly if more people participated in early detection programs. A combination of regular self-exams and screenings provides the best means of detecting cancer early enough to allow for effective treatment. Unfortunately, too many people ignore or are not informed of the recommendations about regular self-exams and screenings.

At present, the American Cancer Society recommends the following screening tests:

- Colon cancer screening: Adults 50 years of age and older should have annual stool testing for occult blood, and either a colonoscopy every 10 years, a flexible sigmoidoscopy every five years, or a double-contrast barium enema every five years.
- Breast cancer screening: Women should have an annual mammogram starting at 40 years of age and scheduled annual breast exams augmented by frequent self-breast exams.
- Cervical cancer screening: Women should have pelvic examinations and PAP smears starting three years after their first sexual encoun-

ter or at 21 years of age. Women 70 years of age or older with more than three normal PAP tests in a row and no abnormal PAP test results in the last 10 years may choose to stop having cervical cancer screening.

• Prostate cancer screening: Men over 50 years of age should consider annual digital-rectal examination and PSA screening.

For each of these screening recommendations, high-risk persons should begin screening at an earlier age.

Some people fail to participate in regular screenings for cancer because of their fear of the pain or indignities associated with the screenings. Therefore, accurate information about the nature of the screenings and the definite benefits of early detection needs to be provided. Special efforts are needed to increase the number of African Americans and Hispanics who participate in early detection programs. Historically, lower rates of participation among minority groups have resulted in later detection of cancers and higher mortality rates than among non-Hispanic whites.

The American Cancer Society developed the mnemonic C-A-U-T-I-O-N as an outline for recognizing common warning signs of cancer:

Change in bowel or bladder habits

A sore that does not heal

Unusual bleeding or discharge

Thickening or lump in the breast or elsewhere

Indigestion or difficulty swallowing

Obvious change in a wart or mole

Nagging cough or hoarseness

These signs and symptoms are not definite indicators of cancer; they can be caused by other problems. However, if they persist for more than two weeks, it is wise to see a physician.

People also need to be aware that their risk of developing cancer may be reduced by making modifications in their lifestyle—most important of which is smoking cessation. The American Cancer Society estimates that more than 80 percent of lung cancer deaths result from smoking and that almost 175,000 cancer deaths each year can be attributed to the use of tobacco. However, even longtime smokers who quit have a reduced risk (compared with people who continue smoking) of lung, laryngeal, esophageal, oral, pancreatic, bladder, and cervical cancer.

Diet can play an important role in reducing the incidence of cancer. High-fat or low-fiber diets may play a causative role in cancer, whereas the daily consumption of vegetables and fruits is associated with a lower risk of lung, prostate, bladder, esophageal, and stomach cancers.

Many people do not realize that the chance of getting cancer increases with age. For example, breast cancer is thought by many to be a disease that primarily affects middle-aged women; in fact, the incidence of breast cancer rises steadily with age, and more than half of women who develop breast cancer do so after 65 years of age. Therefore, it is important for older women to have regular physical examinations and mammograms. Similarly, more than half of the cases of colon cancer, a disease that affects both women and men, occur after 70 years of age.

HOW CAN CANCER BE TREATED?

Many people believe that there are no effective treatments for most types of cancer or that the available treatments are worse than the disease. Consequently, it is important that they be given honest, accurate information about treatments and their right to choose treatments. Patients should be encouraged to ask their physicians about treatment options, the risks and side effects as well as the expected benefits of the treatments, and the consequences of no treatment. The approaches to cancer treatment are increasingly complex and require the expertise of oncologists or even oncology specialists—physicians who gain expertise in caring for a limited number of cancer types. Treatment modalities are diverse and can include infusion of intravenous medications (usually called chemotherapy), oral drugs, radiation therapy, hormonal suppression therapy (e.g., for breast and prostate cancers), and, increasingly, biologic agents engineered to treat a specific cancer. The side effects of treatment also require great attention, and multidisciplinary cancer programs should have expertise in ensuring that these adverse consequences are minimized.

Support groups can be helpful to those with cancer and to their families and friends. They can provide valuable emotional support, and there is evidence that cancer patients who participate in support groups live longer.

SUGGESTIONS FOR CONGREGATIONAL PROGRAMS

Provide education on available screening tests focused on the techniques and technology employed, and the "difficulty" associated with having the test done. Individuals who have had a recent screening test are sometimes the best advocates in allaying the fear others have about being tested.

Arrange for cancer screenings. Some hospitals have mobile mammography units that can be sent to your community. If such a unit is not available, you may be able to arrange transportation to the local hospital for members of your congregation. Screening programs for colorectal cancer making use of mail-in cards to test for occult blood in stool can be distributed for use at home. Local dermatologists might volunteer to do skin cancer screenings. Check with your community hospital to find out the easiest way to provide these screenings for members of your congregation and community.

Provide classes on "Eating and Exercise for a Healthy Life." Both a better diet and more physical activity are associated with lower cancer rates.

Provide help for members of your congregation and community who want to stop smoking. You could either inform them about smoking cessation programs offered in your community or sponsor a class held in one of your congregation's facilities. You can obtain information about programs and materials from your local hospital, the American Lung Association, and the American Cancer Society.

Distribute screening and cancer-related materials to specific groups within your congregation. For example, give information on breast cancer to women's groups and information on prostate cancer to men's groups.

Distribute information on skin cancer and sun exposure to all age groups. Make a special effort to reach children, teenagers, and young adults in the congregation since early sun damage and regular tanning are likely causes of later-life skin cancers. You may wish to emphasize this topic during the spring and summer months.

Sponsor a special program on cancer. An oncologist or medical professional who is regularly involved in the diagnosis or treatment of cancer can serve as your featured speaker. The American Cancer Society can provide materials to distribute at this program.

Sponsor or help members of your congregation find a support group for people who have cancer. Potential leaders for a support group include hospital social workers, mental health professionals, nurses, and cancer survivors. The local hospital and the American Cancer Society can help you locate existing groups or identify qualified group leaders.

EXAMPLES OF CONGREGATIONAL PROGRAMS

An excellent congregational program on cancer was coordinated by Barbara Pearson, a lay health educator who has led a vibrant health ministry at College Park Baptist Church in Orlando, Florida, for more than thirteen years. She asked Dr. Rebecca Moroose, the oncologist who had spoken to her lay health educator class at Florida Hospital, to speak to members of her congregation about cancer. She specifically requested that she address the nature of cancer, how to prevent it, and how to treat it. Dr. Moroose opened with a general overview of cancer, then focused on breast cancer for the rest of her presentation. She used slides to illustrate some of the breast cancers she has treated. The slides were disturbing, but Dr. Moroose, Barbara, and Dr. Charles Horton, the pastor, had agreed in advance that the audience needed to see these pictures. The presentation, including the slides, clearly held the people's attention. The many questions asked by the audience provided evidence of the high level of interest in the topic of cancer and the need for accurate information to dispel some of the common misconceptions about the disease. Most of the people in the audience picked up some of the American Cancer Society materials that had been brought to the meeting by Barbara, and many took the time to thank her for arranging this presentation.

The health ministry team of First Baptist Church of New Smyrna Beach, Florida, led by Betty Severance, a retired nurse, offers many programs for those who face health-related challenges. For example, they provide transportation for individuals who are unable to drive and meals for those who are unable to prepare their own. They also sponsor a quarterly health forum where as many as two hundred come to hear health professionals speak on various topics, including cardiovascular disease, cancer, diabetes, hypertension, depression, nutrition, and exercise. One program has special meaning for Betty—the cancer support group. A cancer survivor herself, Betty knows the many challenges facing individuals with this disease. She initially had been involved in the American Cancer Society's "I Can Cope" program designed for individuals who have been recently diagnosed with cancer. She found that many of the people who completed this course felt a need to continue meeting with others who were facing similar challenges. To address this need, she organized monthly "dialogue" meetings where cancer survivors could come together to share their experiences and feelings. Within this group were individuals who expressed a desire to have a support group that was tied to their religious beliefs and practices. This led Betty to organize a support group at her church that has adopted the name "Christian Cancer Conquerors." The group, usually numbering about fifteen, meets monthly at First Baptist Church and is open to all who are interested. Often there will be a brief presentation by a health professional, but they are careful to always allow time for both open discussion of their concerns and prayer.

INFORMATION RESOURCES

Much of the information and many of the materials needed for your programs can be obtained from your local chapter of the American Cancer Society (ACS) or the organization's Web site (www.cancer.org). To locate the nearest chapter, call 1-800-ACS-2345 (1-800-227-2345) or visit their Web site.

The American Cancer Society or your local hospital can also help you identify professionals, volunteers, and other organizations in your community that can offer services such as guest speakers for community programs, support groups for cancer patients and families, trained cancer survivors who can offer support and information for patients, assistance with transportation and supplies, and smoking cessation classes.

The American Cancer Society sponsors public awareness campaigns and special events throughout the year. Information about the events in your area can be found by visiting the ACS Web site.

The following Internet Web sites also provide information on cancer:

www.cancer.gov (National Cancer Institute)
www.cdc.gov/cancer (Centers for Disease Control and Prevention)
www.cancer.net (American Society of Clinical Oncology)
www.lungusa.org (American Lung Association)
www.komen.org (Susan G. Komen for the Cure)

7

DIABETES MELLITUS

Data from the Centers for Disease Control and Prevention indicate that approximately 24 million Americans (nearly 8% of the U.S. population) have diabetes mellitus, a condition defined by abnormally high levels of glucose (a natural sugar) in the blood. However, almost a quarter of these people do not know they have this serious medical condition. Among people 60 years of age and older, the prevalence is estimated at 25 percent having diabetes mellitus. The prevalence rates are even higher among African Americans and Hispanics and for all adults who are overweight. Besides those with diabetes, more than 55 million other Americans have "prediabetes," or evidence of problems controlling glucose levels that increases their risk of developing diabetes.

There are two major types of diabetes mellitus. Type 1 diabetes, also known as insulin-dependent diabetes mellitus, juvenile diabetes, and brittle diabetes, accounts for approximately 10 percent of all cases. This type is most likely to affect those under 20 years of age, although it can occur at older ages. More common is type 2 diabetes mellitus, also referred to as non–insulin-dependent diabetes mellitus or adult-onset diabetes, generally found in individuals over 40 years of age. Type 2 diabetes accounts for approximately 90 percent of all cases. Although the majority of people with type 2 diabetes are overweight, even lean adults can be affected. Given the epidemic of obesity in the United States, it is now common to find children, adolescents, and adults less than 40 years of age with type 2 diabetes—a situation almost unheard of just a few decades ago.

In persons with diabetes, high blood glucose (hyperglycemia) occurs because there is a breakdown in the normal process of glucose being transported into the body's cells. Insulin, a hormone produced by the pancreas, plays a critical role in the movement of glucose or sugar from the bloodstream into the cells. High levels of blood glucose result when the pancreas does not produce enough insulin (type 1 diabetes) or when the cells are resistant or unresponsive to insulin (type 2 diabetes).

Type 1 diabetes usually develops rapidly, with individuals experiencing unexplained weight loss, frequent urination, and excessive thirst. Sometimes diabetic ketoacidosis, a potentially life-threatening condition with symptoms that include nausea, vomiting, slow respirations, and mental confusion, can be the presenting illness for persons with type 1 diabetes. Type 2 diabetes develops more gradually, and many individuals experience few or no symptoms for several years. Increased thirst and urination can be seen, along with visual disturbances or even fungal rashes of the feet or groin. Occasionally, individuals with type 2 diabetes develop ketoacidosis under certain circumstances, but the more serious problems associated with type 2 diabetes are its long-term complications.

WHO IS AT RISK?

It is important that people at high risk for developing diabetes have the appropriate screening tests. At least two screening tests separated by a few days or weeks must be abnormal to make and confirm the diagnosis of diabetes. (Sometimes diet, medications, or illness can lead to an elevated blood glucose measurement in those who do not have diabetes and therefore having a second test is a necessary step in diagnosis.) The two most common tests are the fasting glucose and oral glucose tolerance tests. For the fasting glucose test, the patient fasts overnight for at least ten hours, blood is drawn and tested the next morning, and the glucose value over 126 mg/dl is consistent with a diagnosis of diabetes. For an oral glucose tolerance test, the same procedure as for a fasting glucose test is initially followed. But in addition, after the first blood is drawn, the patient drinks a sugary mixture and has a second blood sample drawn two hours later. If the fasting blood glucose is over 126 mg/dl or if the blood glucose two hours later is over 200 mg/dl, a diagnosis of diabetes can be made.

Persons at risk for developing diabetes include everyone over 45 years of age, those with a family member who has diabetes, Asian Americans, African Americans, Hispanics, Native Americans, Pacific Islanders, people who are overweight or obese, women with previous gestational diabetes (or diabetes diagnosed while pregnant) or with babies born weighing more than nine pounds, and women with a diagnosis of polycystic ovarian disease.

People who are at risk for diabetes must advocate for themselves and ask their health care providers to order the appropriate screening tests.

THE RISKS OF IGNORING INFORMATION ON DIABETES

The millions of people who have diabetes but are not receiving treatment are at risk for many of the chronic complications of diabetes. Undetected and untreated diabetes sets the stage for other diseases or conditions that can kill or cripple:

- Stroke. Older adults with diabetes are almost twice as likely as those without diabetes to have a stroke.
- Heart disease. Older adults with diabetes are at least twice as likely to develop cardiovascular disease, and heart attacks are more likely to be fatal.
- Amputation. The risk of lower-extremity amputation is ten times greater for older adults with diabetes.
- Eye disease. Cataracts, glaucoma, and retinopathy (damage to the retina) are more common among older adults with diabetes.
- Kidney disease. Approximately 20 percent of individuals with type 2 diabetes develop nephropathy (kidney damage) that often leads to kidney failure and the need for dialysis.

WHAT CAN BE DONE TO PREVENT DIABETES?

There are no tests or interventions currently recognized that can identify those at risk for or that can prevent the development of type 1 diabetes. Fortunately, the development of type 1 diabetes occurs much less frequently than type 2 diabetes, and individuals at risk for type 2 diabetes are easy to identify. Since obesity and inactivity are the two most potent risk factors for developing type 2 diabetes, those who are overweight and inactive should undergo regular screening tests to check blood glucose. Such testing can identify "pre-diabetes" and provide an early warning sign and impetus to spur meaningful lifestyle changes to prevent the progression to diabetes. Those who lose weight and become more active are less likely to develop type 2 diabetes. In fact, even among individuals who are overweight, regular exercise can improve glucose control and thereby likely postpone the development of diabetes even without weight loss. Thus, the best way to prevent type 2 diabetes is through weight control and exercise.

If either type 1 or type 2 diabetes is detected, some of the long-term complications can be eliminated or their severity greatly reduced with treatment. Although treatment of type 1 diabetes includes daily injections of insulin, many cases of type 2 diabetes do not require insulin injections. There are now a number of ways to administer insulin, including use of an inhaler or a pump. (An insulin pump is a small pager-like device worn on the waistband or belt that is programmed to deliver insulin through an attached catheter or thin plastic tube inserted under the skin.) Type 2 diabetes often can be controlled through diet, weight control, and exercise. Oral medications may be needed if diet and exercise do not adequately control glucose levels. Some persons with type 2 diabetes will require insulin therapy to control the blood glucose levels. Insulin therapy should not be viewed as a punishment, but as an important medication that can accomplish the important goal of returning the high blood glucose levels to near normal levels.

Although it may seem that people who are diagnosed with type 2 diabetes have a relatively simple treatment regimen to follow, many find it difficult to follow their doctor's recommendations consistently. It is not easy to make major lifestyle changes, especially when there are no immediately noticeable consequences. Changes in established patterns are difficult to make and even more difficult to maintain; therefore, patients need the ongoing encouragement and support of family and friends. Ultimately, it is achieving the best glucose control through diet, exercise, oral medications, and/or insulin therapy that will avoid the major complications of diabetes.

SUGGESTIONS FOR CONGREGATIONAL PROGRAMS

Sponsor glucose level testing by working with representatives from the local hospital's medical laboratory or another community medical laboratory. If these representatives cannot conduct the testing at your facility, perhaps you can arrange for transportation to their facility.

Sponsor a special program on diabetes with a physician, nurse educator, or dietitian as your featured speaker. Provide snacks appropriate for people with diabetes.

Offer a support group for patients and families affected by diabetes. Support groups can assist patients in complying with treatment recommendations and also in coping with some of the emotional challenges often associated with diabetes. Your hospital or the American Diabetes Association can assist you in establishing a support group or in locating support groups in the community.

Sponsor or help members of your congregation locate exercise and weight-reduction programs. Most people find it easier to sustain their exercise or weight reduction efforts if they are a part of a group.

Offer cooking classes for patients and families affected by diabetes. A hospital dietitian or the American Diabetes Association can assist with materials and other resources for this program.

Use congregational bulletins and mailings to provide members with basic information on diabetes. This information can be obtained from many sources, including materials available from the American Diabetes Association. Your local chapter may be able to provide copies of brochures and booklets for distribution to your members.

Use church bulletins and mailings to provide members with regular reminders about monitoring their glucose level and complying with treatment recommendations.

EXAMPLES OF CONGREGATIONAL PROGRAMS

The **S**creening, **T**eaching, **E**xercise, and **P**revention (S.T.E.P.) program offered by Seton Health's Faith Community Nursing program in Troy, New York, is a good example of how religious congregations and medical institutions can work together to address the problem of diabetes. This program, led by Fran Zoske, M.S.N., R.N., director of Seton Health Faith Community

Nursing Program and associate professor of nursing at Empire State College, is modeled after the successful Spring into Healthy Habits program held at several churches that are engaged in cooperative partnerships with St. John Community Health of Warren, Michigan. Both health systems are a part of Ascension Health, the nation's largest Catholic nonprofit health system.

The S.T.E.P. on Diabetes program identifies individuals at risk for developing diabetes and provides educational programs aimed at decreasing risk factors while increasing healthy lifestyles. Participants are reached through Seton Health's Faith Community Nursing Program and six of the churches they serve in the New York communities of Troy, Waterford, and Clifton Park. Screenings and assessments take place at these churches. Screening activities include an initial paper and pencil risk test, finger stick for blood glucose and lipid panel, blood pressure check, and measurement of height, weight, body mass index, and waist circumference. Individuals found to possibly have undiagnosed diabetes are referred to primary care physicians, with referral arrangements in place for those who are uninsured or underinsured. Individuals who are identified as being at risk for developing diabetes are encouraged to attend a series of four classes entitled "Healthy Living." These classes focus on setting goals for healthier lifestyles, increasing physical activity, eating nutritiously, lowering stress, and identifying emotional eating habits. Once the Healthy Living classes have ended, additional educational programs and support groups are provided by the faith community nurses within the churches. Follow-up assessments are conducted in conjunction with the Healthy Living classes and during monthly support group sessions.

Spring into Healthy Habits, the program that provided the inspiration for the S.T.E.P. program, was supported by a grant received by St. John Community Health in 2004. This grant was to support programming targeting African Americans, with the objective of improving minority health. Partnerships were developed between St. John Community Health and local churches to screen, educate, and engage members in exercise. The grant provided support for a period of two and a half years and resulted in the screening of more than a thousand people. The class format generated enthusiasm, and the evaluation showed that the majority of participants had learned new information about how to lower their risks and had implemented their personal goals. Specifically, analysis of the data revealed significant changes in body mass index, waist circumference, and patient empowerment scores. Ongoing relationships with the faith communities provide St. John with the ability to continue the education and risk reduction program after the completion of the grant.

The Seton Health S.T.E.P. program was awarded a $500,000 grant from New York State in January 2008 to further expand their program as well as to identify best practices in diabetes management and prevention. This grant involves a multifaceted approach using physicians, diabetes educators, faith community nurses, and a computer-based registry. It is anticipated that this multifaceted approach will provide evidence-based results necessary to determine a best practice approach to diabetes management that can be further replicated throughout the state.

Another example of the value of a congregational program on diabetes is offered by Dr. Annabelle Rodriguez, a Johns Hopkins endocrinologist who consulted with us on this chapter:

As an endocrinologist, I had thought for some time that it might be easier to spread the word about diabetes in an informal atmosphere, such as in a church setting, than to give lectures in a formal presentation. I approached a patient, a pastor who had diabetes, and told her of my interest.

Pastor G.W. readily agreed to allow me to meet with members of her parish one Sunday afternoon. I arrived around 2:00 p.m., and did not leave until close to 4:00 p.m. Admittedly, this first meeting was a bit awkward, as I did not have the comfort of slides and a laser pointer, and the church parishioners were not sure of the intent of the meeting. But the awkwardness did not last long. I said that my intent was to offer a forum by which they could ask me anything regarding diabetes, and soon a spirited dialogue began.

The first question was: "What's an endocrinologist?" That question then sparked a number of follow-up questions. Although the first meeting was only attended by a handful of individuals, over the subsequent months the group grew larger, with children and grandparents in attendance. All the questions were inquisitive and insightful.

For me, one of the most memorable experiences came when members formed a walking group, and they reported significant weight loss and improvement in their blood sugar and blood pressure. They were always interested in how to make healthy food choices. For instance, many reported making the switch from high-sugar breakfast cereals to ones higher in fiber content.

On professional and personal levels, it was gratifying to impart health care information in an atmosphere that was comforting and welcoming both to the church members and to me. I am certain that fostering these types of alliances are of major benefit to the community at large.

INFORMATION RESOURCES

Your local chapter of the American Diabetes Association can provide much of the information and many of the materials you will need for your programs. You can locate the nearest office of the American Diabetes Association by visiting their Web site (www.diabetes.org) or calling 1-800-DIABETES (1-800-342-2383). The American Diabetes Association or your local hospital can also help you identify professionals, volunteers, and other organizations in your community that offer services such as guest speakers for congregational and community programs, support groups for patients with diabetes and their families, educational classes (e.g., nutrition) for patients with diabetes and their families, and information on medical supplies.

The American Diabetes Association sponsors a national diabetes awareness campaign every November. You may wish to schedule a congregational program on diabetes to coincide with this national campaign.

The following Web sites also provide information on diabetes:

www.niddk.nih.gov (National Institute of Diabetes and Digestive and Kidney Diseases)
www.cdc.gov/diabetes (Centers for Disease Control and Prevention)

8

DEPRESSION

Depression, a serious condition that affects millions of Americans every year, is different from the periods of sadness or feelings of grief that occur as an expected part of life for most people. Although it is normal to be sad or "down" occasionally and to experience grief when a significant loss occurs, clinical depression has more severe symptoms, often sustained over a long period of time, and is more likely to affect an individual's ability to function normally.

It is estimated that during any given month almost 5 percent of Americans will experience an episode of major depression. The lifetime chance of having a major depression is more than 17 percent. When other depressive conditions such as bipolar and dysthymic disorders are included, the estimate of lifetime prevalence exceeds 20 percent. In other words, one of every five Americans will experience at least one serious episode of depression at some point during his or her life. Females are approximately twice as likely as males to experience an episode of major depression. Recent studies indicate that depression is increasing among the young and the old, with younger age cohorts more likely to experience depression than older ones.

Depression is not only painful but can also greatly impair a person's relationships and ability to work productively. In many cases it is a life-threatening condition, placing people at risk for death from suicide or physical conditions such as heart disease.

One of the most unfortunate and tragic aspects of depression is that in spite of the availability of several effective methods of treatment, it frequently goes undetected and untreated. Often the symptoms are incorrectly attributed to medical conditions or other factors—particularly aging. Even when people are aware of their depression, they may underestimate the seriousness of the disorder or feel hopeless about finding effective treatment. Many people, especially elderly individuals, do not view depression as a serious condition that may require professional help; they believe that they are responsible for bringing on the depression and that only they can "remove" their depression.

Because depression is so frequently undetected, it is important for congregational health education programs to inform their members about the symptoms of depression. These are the most common symptoms:

Depressed mood with sustained feelings of sadness and grief
Loss of interest and pleasure in activities formerly enjoyed
Insomnia, early morning waking, or oversleeping nearly every day
Decreased energy, fatigue, end-of-day exhaustion
Noticeable changes in appetite and weight (a significant loss or gain)
Feelings of guilt, worthlessness, and helplessness
Indecisiveness or an inability to concentrate or think
Recurrent thoughts of death and suicide
Restlessness or slowing down

An episode of major depression is diagnosed when a person has experienced five or more of these symptoms every day or almost every day during a two-week period. At least one of the symptoms must be depressed mood or loss of interest or pleasure in activities previously enjoyed.

Another form of depression is dysthymic disorder. This is a milder but chronic pattern of depression. People with this disorder experience symptoms of depression almost every day for at least two years. During this period, they are almost never without the symptoms of depression for more than two months. In addition to depressed mood, they experience two or more of the following symptoms:

Poor appetite or overeating
Insomnia or hypersomnia
Low energy or fatigue

Low self-esteem
Poor concentration or difficulty making decisions
Feelings of hopelessness

A third mood disorder in which a person experiences episodes of depression is bipolar disorder (also known as manic-depressive disorder). In addition to the depression, the person experiences mania or hypomania. Symptoms of mania or hypomania are:

Inflated self-esteem or grandiosity
Decreased need for sleep
Unusual need to talk more or feelings of pressure to keep talking
Flight of ideas or subjective experience that thoughts are racing
Distractibility
Increase in goal-directed activity or psychomotor agitation
Excessive involvement in pleasurable activities that have a high
    potential for adverse consequences

In the case of a manic episode, at least three of these symptoms persist for at least one week and are severe enough to impair significantly occupational or social functioning. In the case of hypomania, the symptoms persist for at least four days but do not significantly impair occupational or social functioning.

The primary reason that it is important to note whether a depression is accompanied by symptoms of mania or hypomania is that bipolar disorders require different treatment from that typically used for unipolar or major depression and dysthymic disorder. Specifically, antidepressants can worsen manic symptoms and are therefore often avoided for people who have bipolar disorder.

THE RISKS OF IGNORING INFORMATION
ON DEPRESSION

The most serious consequence of failing to detect and treat depression is the greatly increased risk of suicide. The suicide rate increases with age and is highest among older men. The tremendous emotional pain, combined with the sense of hopelessness about ever obtaining relief from the pain, leads many depressed people to see death as their only escape.

Because of the harmful effects of depression on the immune system and the feelings of hopelessness and helplessness associated with depression, depressed people are more likely to experience other health problems and suffer more harmful consequences from existing physical illnesses. For example, someone who has a heart attack and is depressed is more likely to die than someone who has a heart attack but is not depressed. In addition, depressed people are less likely to follow the treatment recommendations for their other conditions and diseases. Depressed people are more likely to develop diabetes, and depressed people who have diabetes have more trouble managing their blood sugar.

The emotional and financial costs of depression often go well beyond the depressed person. Depression can contribute to marital and family conflict, work impairment, and financial problems. Too frequently we read accounts in the newspaper of destructive or deadly actions that were caused at least in part by depression.

WHAT CAN BE DONE TO PREVENT DEPRESSION?

The first step to be taken in any congregational program on depression is to increase the members' ability to recognize this disorder. Depression often goes undetected because we attribute some of the symptoms to other factors. We call this the *trap of meaning*—a meaningful explanation is given to symptoms caused by a brain dysfunction. For example, we may not be surprised when a teenager seems moody and withdraws from family and friends. We may assume that this is typical and does not call for any special attention. Depression can also be especially difficult to detect among the elderly. Older adults are less likely to report that they are depressed, and often the symptoms of depression are attributed to physical disorders or are thought to be a normal part of aging. Also, people with dementia have different symptoms when they are depressed—mostly loss of interest, anxiousness, irritability, and often delusions. Because of these difficulties in detecting depression, a health education program needs to find creative ways to distribute information so that people can recognize the symptoms of depression in themselves and others.

The second step is to give people hope about their treatment for depression. There are several effective biological and psychological treatments. People with depression are not doomed to a life of misery if they seek professional help, but many fail to ask for help. Why? One reason is the stigma that many people still feel is attached to depression or any mental disorder. They believe that it is a sign of weakness or moral failure. Many believe that if only their faith were stronger, they would not be depressed. Because of these beliefs, they are embarrassed to let others know they are depressed. These beliefs can constitute a serious and dangerous barrier to treatment. A congregational health education program must find ways to eliminate this barrier.

The third step is to give the congregation reliable, up-to-date information on treatment options. They should learn about both biological and psychological methods. Currently, many effective medications are available. The antidepressant medications that have been around the longest are available generically (e.g., amitriptyline and nortriptyline), and are still recognized as effective in relieving depression. Several newer antidepressant drugs (e.g., Zoloft, Paxil, and Prozac) also are now available in generic form, and these have fewer side effects. This point is a particularly important consideration because many people will stop taking medications if they produce unpleasant side effects. All antidepressant medications should result in significant improvement in symptoms within six weeks. While most of these medications can be prescribed by a family physician or internist, treatment by a psychiatrist is often appropriate and necessary when symptoms are severe or if response to treatment is delayed and changes in antidepressants are being considered to restore normal levels of mood and functioning.

Most of the psychological therapies that have been demonstrated to be effective in the treatment of depression (e.g., cognitive behavioral therapy, interpersonal therapy, and dialectical behavioral therapy) are relatively short-term and focused. They do not involve years of treatment or a detailed examination of childhood issues. In fact, psychotherapy should produce noticeable improvement within six weeks. Psychological treatment in combination with antidepressant medication is especially effective in relieving depression.

Electroconvulsive therapy (ECT) has been demonstrated to be an effective treatment for certain types of severe depression that do not respond to other forms of treatment. Because it is administered under anesthesia, ECT is not the barbaric treatment it once appeared to be. Patients do not experience pain during the treatments, and their bodies do not shake or jerk. Although there may be short-term confusion after each treatment, there are seldom any signs of memory problems two to three weeks after the treatments are completed, and there is no long-term memory loss or brain damage.

The fourth step is to inform the congregation about the risk of suicide among those suffering from depression. Suicides occur among all age groups, but suicide rates are highest among older adults, especially males. Often these suicides are related to a personal or family illness. Among teenagers, suicide is one of the leading killers, and recent studies show an increase in the number of suicides for the 5–19 age group. Suicides among teenagers and young adults are frequently linked to problems in relationships.

Finally, the congregational program on depression should provide guidance and support for individuals who have loved ones who are depressed. It can be especially challenging to try to care for persons who no longer find pleasure in any of the activities they previously enjoyed and who are thoroughly pessimistic about ever feeling better. The National Institute of Mental Health (NIMH) offers the following suggestions for families and friends:

- Help him or her get an appropriate diagnosis and treatment. You may need to make an appointment on behalf of your friend or relative and go with him or her to see the doctor.
- Encourage him or her to stay in treatment or to seek different treatment if no improvement occurs after six to eight weeks.
- Offer emotional support, understanding, patience, and encouragement.
- Never disparage feelings your friend or relative expresses, but point out realities and offer hope.
- Never ignore comments about suicide, and report them to your friend's or relative's therapist or doctor.
- Invite your friend or relative out for walks, outings, and other activi-

ties. Keep trying if he or she declines, but don't push him or her to take on too much too soon. Although diversions and company are needed, too many demands may increase feelings of failure.

• Remind your friend or relative that with time and treatment the depression will lift.

SUGGESTIONS FOR CONGREGATIONAL PROGRAMS

Raise your congregation's awareness of depression by placing information on the symptoms, prevalence, and treatment of depression in congregational bulletins and mailings. Special attention should be given to the encouraging news about effective treatments for depression. Materials on these topics can be obtained from the National Institute of Mental Health, Mental Health America, the Depression and Bipolar Support Alliance, and the National Alliance on Mental Illness.

Reduce the stigma attached to depression by having respected leaders of your congregation emphasize that depression is a common disorder that does not reflect weakness or moral failure. It should be recognized and treated as a medical condition, not as a character flaw. The personal testimony of an individual who has experienced depression and knows the definite benefits of medical and psychological treatments can be especially effective.

Provide members of your congregation with information about support groups and other services available to people encountering stressful experiences (e.g., marital separation or divorce, chronic illnesses). If there are no support groups in your community, your congregation may wish to help organize and sponsor one.

Sponsor a class on pain management for individuals experiencing chronic pain. Physicians and psychologists who specialize in pain management can teach strategies and skills that can help people reduce their pain and give them greater independence. Your hospital or an agency specializing in rehabilitation medicine should be able to help you locate a professional to teach the class.

Offer a special program on antidepressant medications. A physician or pharmacist can provide information that can allay some of the fears and correct misconceptions about these medications. One specific issue that should be addressed is the need for people to take the medications as prescribed. Too often patients fail to understand and follow doctors' recommendations.

Incorporate information on depression into regularly scheduled programs and activities. Many of the people who need information on depression may be reluctant to attend a special program on the subject. They may feel more comfortable if this information is provided in regularly scheduled programs.

Arrange for a mental health professional to provide training for congregational leaders who teach classes or who have responsibility for visiting members so that these individuals can learn how to check for symptoms of depression. This will enable the leaders to determine whether members who decrease their participation in congregational activities they previously enjoyed could be suffering from depression.

Find opportunities for discussions on suicide among the various age groups in your congregation. This topic needs to be addressed openly. People need to learn that the hopelessness expressed by depressed persons often leads to suicide.

Publish in congregational bulletins and mailings the telephone numbers of the local suicide hotline and other agencies where a person in distress can call or visit if he or she needs immediate assistance.

Encourage people to read first-person accounts to obtain a better understanding of the depressive experience and help them see that even intelligent, successful people can have depression. Three books that can be recommended are *Darkness Visible,* by William Styron; *Undercurrents,* by Martha Manning, Ph.D.; and *An Unquiet Mind,* by Kay Redfield Jamison, Ph.D. Additional information on these books is provided under the suggested readings section.

EXAMPLES OF CONGREGATIONAL PROGRAMS

I (WDH) am frequently invited by congregations to give a presentation on depression, a topic that has interested me since graduate school and that has been the focus of much of my research and clinical work over the years. When I began giving these presentations, the invitations were often accompanied by a cautionary comment from congregational leaders reflecting their concern that a program on depression might not draw as large an audience as programs on other health topics. I quickly discovered that they should not have been worried about poor attendance. In fact, in almost every congregation, attendance for the program on depression was as high as or even higher than that for programs on heart disease, hypertension, diabetes, and other strictly medical topics. Furthermore, people were interested in all aspects of depression: How can one recognize it? What medications and psychological treatments are effective? How can people help loved ones who suffer from depression? What should one do if a friend or family member might be suicidal?

Although for most of my presentations I have spoken from the perspective of a clinical psychologist who has been involved in the diagnosis and treatment of depression, there have been occasions when I have felt it was appropriate to also talk about what it was like when I became seriously depressed in my late thirties. One of the reasons I have at times shared my personal experience is to help remove or at least diminish the stigma that is all too often still attached to depression. Although there is greater openness about depression today than there was ten or twenty years ago, there are still many people reluctant to speak as openly about depression as they would about hypertension or diabetes. It is important for health professionals and religious leaders to do whatever we can to remove the stigma attached to depression and other mental illnesses, and one way is for me to be open about my own experience. The other reason I have talked about my depressive episode is to help people understand how painful and debilitating the experience can be and how hopeless everything can seem, but also how there are effective treatments for depression and how the support of family and friends is important when one is in the depths of a depression.

A few weeks after one of my presentations at which I had discussed my own experience with depression, I received a note from a woman who had attended my talk. She wrote that her attendance at this program marked the first time she had been in her church in several months. She had stayed away, she said, because she felt so utterly worthless and that there was nothing at all in her life for which she felt thankful and nothing to look forward to. It would feel "wrong" for her to be in her church where others seemed so full of joy and hope, and she was certain other people would not want to be around her. But when she received the church newsletter and read that there would be a program on depression, she decided to make the effort to attend. She went on to say that it was during my presentation that she first began to see at least a little ray of hope about her situation. If someone else had felt as bad as she did and then had gone on to recover and return to an active, fulfilling life, perhaps she could too. And the encouraging information about the benefits of antidepressant medication and psychotherapy gave her further hope.

Armed with the information about treatments for depression, she had made an appointment with her family physician, who agreed that she was depressed and prescribed medication. Her physician had also referred her to a psychologist known for her work with depressed individuals. She concluded by saying that with the help of the medication and her therapist, she had begun to emerge from her depression and was on her way back to being the sociable and confident person she had been before sinking into her depression.

Another informative congregational program on depression took place one Friday evening following the Shabbat service at Temple Beth El in Ormond Beach, Florida. At the end of the service, Rabbi Barry Altman introduced Dr. Maximo Handel, a psychiatrist, who spoke for about fifteen minutes on many important aspects of depression. He described the symptoms, causal factors, and some of the treatments that are available. He pointed out that depression is a treatable condition but that often persons suffering from depression feel so hopeless and helpless that they fail to realize there are effective treatments available. He also pointed out that family members frequently fail to detect the signs of depression or attribute them to other causes. Dr. Handel emphasized the great importance of recognizing and treating depression because of the extreme pain and suffering it causes the affected individual, the detrimental impact it can have on relationships and work, and the increased risk of suicide. At the conclusion of the presentation, Rabbi Altman joined him and encouraged members of the congregation to ask questions about depression and other mental disorders. After a few questions, Rabbi Altman invited others who had questions to speak with Dr. Handel at the Oneg that followed the service, and several members of the congregation used this opportunity to speak with him about personal concerns.

INFORMATIONAL RESOURCES

Your local affiliate of Mental Health America (formerly known as the National Mental Health Association) can provide many of the materials you can use in your programs as well as information about other resources in your community (e.g., screenings and referrals, guest speakers for community programs, support groups for depressed persons and their families, support groups for persons going through various stressful experiences). You can locate the nearest affiliate by visiting the Web site for Mental Health America (www.nmha.org) or calling 1-800-969-6642.

Information and materials appropriate for use in congregational programs also can be obtained from

www.nimh.nih.gov (National Institute of Mental Health)

www.ndmda.org – 1-800-826-3632 (Depression and Bipolar Support Alliance)

www.nami.org – 1-800-950-6264 (National Alliance on Mental Illness).

9

DEMENTIA

Dementia is a clinical syndrome or condition in which there is a progressive deterioration of mental faculties, usually over many years. Problems with memory are usually the first sign of dementia. Other symptoms may include difficulties with language, impaired judgment, problems in performing simple tasks such as dressing, and changes in personality and behavior. Most people with dementia also develop clinical depression, agitation, anxiety, or other "behavioral symptoms" as their disease progresses.

Dementia is not an inevitable consequence of aging. Although the risk of dementia increases with age, the overwhelming majority of older adults do not have dementia. It is important to understand that most older adults who report problems with memory do not have and may never develop dementia. Minor problems with memory may be a normal part of aging and should not be viewed as evidence of dementia.

Dementia can be caused by a number of brain disorders. The most common is Alzheimer's disease, which accounts for approximately 50–60 percent of all cases of dementia. Alzheimer's is a progressive, degenerative disease that attacks the brain. There is loss of nerve cells, especially in the regions responsible for memory and intellectual functions. Currently there is no cure for this irreversible disease, although several newer medications can result in modest improvements in mental functions for some affected people.

Dementia resulting from vascular disease is the second most common type. This form of dementia occurs when there is damage to multiple small areas of the brain. This is typically thought to arise as a series of "small strokes" resulting from atherosclerosis and blockage of small arteries in the brain that occur over a period of months or years. For this reason, vascular dementia is now generally referred to as multi-infarct dementia. There are many risk factors for vascular dementia; the most important is hypertension. Individuals can reduce their risk of experiencing this form of dementia by controlling their blood pressure, avoiding smoking, eating a low-fat diet, exercising regularly, and controlling their weight.

Another common condition that can cause the symptoms of dementia, particularly in older adults, is depression. Older depressed individuals often have problems with memory, experience periods of confusion, and can be unresponsive to other people. It is important to distinguish correctly when dementia is caused by depression because effective medical and psychological treatments for depression might reverse the dementia symptoms. Other causes of reversible dementias include overmedication, unusual drug reactions, thyroid disease, and some vitamin deficiencies. Like depression, these can be treated if they are correctly identified.

THE RISKS OF IGNORING INFORMATION ON DEMENTIA

The potential harm of relying on inaccurate or incomplete information about dementia and the health care resources appropriate for managing this condition goes beyond the patient. Dementia is frequently referred to as a "caregiver's disease" because of its tremendous impact on the family. The spouse and other members of the patient's family face many new challenges and stresses that can seem overwhelming and endless. The decisions and pressures the family faces may produce conflict among family members. Also, it is not uncommon for family members to experience depression in reaction to this difficult situation. Family members who confront these challenges without the appropriate knowledge, skills, and resources are in danger of developing their own health problems.

The belief that dementia is inevitable and that there is no effective treatment for any type of dementia can have painful consequences for patients and their families. Patients who are thought to have dementia but who actually are depressed suffer unnecessary pain and limitations, and so do their families.

In addition, the belief that nothing can be done to prevent the development of dementia can have harmful consequences. This belief, frequently based on the mistaken notion that all dementias are the result of

Alzheimer's disease, can become a self-fulfilling prophecy. In fact, several steps can be taken to reduce the risk of experiencing vascular dementia. Furthermore, these same steps may also reduce the risk of developing the symptoms of Alzheimer's disease. Recent studies have shown that some people with the brain abnormalities associated with Alzheimer's disease do not show its symptoms. Researchers found that the memory loss and confusion associated with Alzheimer's disease most likely results from the combination of the brain deterioration of Alzheimer's disease and one or more small strokes in certain regions of the brain.

Although there is no cure for dementia, a lot can be done to help patients and caregivers. The American Association for Geriatric Psychiatry (AAGP) recently published a position statement related to caring for individuals with Alzheimer's disease that reviews the use of medications and nonpharmacologic interventions (e.g., reorientation, cueing, prompts) to treat symptoms, encourages participation in clinical trials of medications under development, and suggests specific activities targeted at caregiver and patient support as critical aspects of care. (See www.aagponline.org/prof/position_caredmnalz.asp.) Several medications (e.g., Aricept, Exelon, and Razadyne) are approved by the U.S. Food and Drug Administration to treat Alzheimer's disease and may improve some of the memory symptoms. Other important treatments for dementia target the psychological and behavioral symptoms such as depression, agitation, sleep problems, delusions, and hallucinations that are frequent in people who have dementia. These include nonmedication interventions (e.g., daily structure, sleep hygiene, behavioral management) and medications (e.g. antidepressants and neuroleptics). The latter should always be used under careful guidance from a specialist because they may carry additional risks for persons with dementia. Supportive care for patients makes sure that they are safe (e.g., through stopping driving, increasing supervision, preventing wandering), that they have a structured daily life plan, and that they are active. Supportive care for caregivers makes sure they are taught caregiving skills, that they are well educated about dementia, and that they have adequate respite.

WHAT CAN BE DONE TO REDUCE
THE IMPACT OF DEMENTIA?

Although there is no cure for most cases of dementia, there are ways to soften its impact on patients and their families. Many families initially wish to keep a loved one with dementia at home, but they soon become overwhelmed by the problems this presents. Families can overcome many of these problems if they have a good understanding of dementia and know some effective strategies. Fortunately, materials and programs are available that can provide families with information about how to better manage the home care of individuals with dementia. Studies have shown that families that learn about dementia and effective management and coping strategies are able to delay placing their loved one in a nursing home almost a year longer than those without similar knowledge and resources.

Many families that are determined to keep their loved one at home become overwhelmed because they fail to use the services of the various agencies and organizations in the community that offer assistance to patients with dementia and their families. Respite care and adult day care programs can provide caregivers with much-needed relief from the seemingly constant demands of monitoring and caring for a cognitively impaired person. Unfortunately, families are often unaware of these services.

Support groups are an important part of the care of patients with dementia and their families. Many of the emotional conflicts and burdens associated with the constant care of a loved one with dementia can be eased by sharing feelings and information with others facing the same challenges.

People also need to become more aware of the encouraging developments in the area of prevention. They need to understand the relationship between dementia and modifiable risk factors such as hypertension.

SUGGESTIONS FOR CONGREGATIONAL PROGRAMS

Sponsor a special program on dementia. A neurologist, psychiatrist, or other physician familiar with dementia can provide helpful information and should be able to respond to the various questions and concerns of the audience. The Mini-Mental State Examination, a brief scoring tool that takes a few minutes for a trained professional to administer, might be reviewed to show how easy the first tests can be in identifying individuals with early cognitive problems. You may wish to provide free blood pressure checks before or after the physician's talk. This will help people make the connection between hypertension and some forms of dementia.

Sponsor a special program on the community resources available to patients and families affected by dementia. This could include information about the various living arrangements appropriate for dementia patients at different stages of their condition. A social worker or case manager from a hospital, nursing home, or home health agency could serve as your featured speaker.

Compile and distribute a list of agencies and organizations in your community that provide services appropriate for patients and families affected by dementia. This could include support groups, respite care programs, adult day care centers, and home health agencies.

Compile and distribute a list of books and materials that offer families advice on managing dementia. One book that should be on this list is *The 36-Hour Day: A Family Guide to Caring for People with Alzheimer Disease, Other Dementias, and Memory Loss in Later Life* (4th ed.), by Nancy L. Mace and Peter V. Rabins. Another monograph, *Practical Dementia Care* (2nd ed.), by Peter V. Rabins, Constantine G. Lyketsos, and Cynthia D. Steele, provides considerable detail for professionals on how to provide dementia care (see suggested readings for more information on these books).

Sponsor a weekly or monthly "Caregivers' Night Out" program. Families that are caring for a loved one who has dementia get few opportunities to meet their own social needs. Even if they are using adult day care, family members usually have to spend their evenings caring for and monitoring their cognitively impaired relative. Most would welcome the opportunity to have an evening to go out if they knew that their afflicted relative was receiving good care arranged by their congregation.

EXAMPLES OF CONGREGATIONAL PROGRAMS

A program co-sponsored by the O'Neill Foundation for Community Health (see chapter 17) and Stetson University in DeLand, Florida, illustrates the high degree of interest within many congregations in the topic of Alzheimer's disease. Congregations in surrounding communities were invited to send representatives to attend a Saturday workshop held on the campus of Stetson University. This workshop featured a video presentation by Dr. Peter Rabins along with a speaker from the Alzheimer's Association. Dr. Rabins, a psychiatrist on the faculty of the Johns Hopkins University School of Medicine, is the co-author of the best-selling book, *The 36-Hour Day*. Fifty-five congregational representatives participated in the program and heard Dr. Rabins address many of the most important aspects of Alzheimer's disease—how it differs from normal aging, how the diagnosis is made, the typical progression of the disease, types of treatments available, the challenges that families will face, and how congregations can be of help to affected individuals and their families. This video presentation was followed by a speaker from the Alzheimer's Association who shared information about local resources. At the conclusion of the program, participants who felt that individuals or groups within their congregation would want to hear this information were given copies of Dr. Rabins's video presentation. Each person taking a copy of the video was asked to estimate how many people were likely to view the video in the next twelve months. When their estimates were totaled, they numbered more than 4,400. A similar program was held at Munroe Regional Medical Center in Ocala, Florida. More than 80 representatives of nearby congregations attended this workshop and received DVDs of Dr. Rabins's presentation. When their estimates of the people who would view the video over the next twelve months were totaled, the number exceeded 7,000.

A good example of a congregational program on the topic of caring for individuals with Alzheimer's disease is one coordinated by lay health educators representing four churches in the greater Daytona Beach area—Grace Episcopal, All Saints Lutheran, Westminster by-the-Sea Presbyterian, and Daytona Beach Christian and Missionary Alliance. The representatives organized an afternoon program on short- and long-term care options for individuals who have dementia or are physically frail. They put together a panel of experts that included a physician who specialized in geriatrics (Dr. Neil Oslos of the Family Practice Residency Program at Halifax Health Medical Center), a discharge planner from a local hospital (Halifax Health Medical Center), the director of an adult day care center, and an administrator from an agency that provided in-home medical and personal care services. Rev. Jeffrey Sumner, the pastor of Westminster by-the-Sea Presbyterian Church, served as the moderator.

Dr. Oslos began the program and touched on many important aspects of medical care for cognitively impaired and physically frail persons. He also explained how factors other than the underlying illness must be considered when searching for long-term care options. For example, the functional abilities (ability to care for oneself) and the availability of a caregiver must be taken into account. The discharge planner then discussed the options she has when helping the patient and family identify the appropriate setting. Next, the director of the adult day care center described the services provided in that type of setting. She also handed out and reviewed a list of the terms frequently used by professionals discussing care options for people with chronic illness. Finally, the administrator of the home health agency shared information on the medical and personal care services his organization could provide.

Rev. Sumner served as the moderator for the question-and-answer part of the program. The questions from the audience revealed that there was great interest in the topic and that many people were unaware of the resources in their community. It was clear that the lay health educators had provided a valuable service by bringing together a group of professionals whose expertise spanned virtually the entire range of issues on the topic of caring for cognitively impaired and physically frail elderly persons.

INFORMATION RESOURCES

Many communities have a chapter of the Alzheimer's Association. You can call the national office of the Alzheimer's Association (1-800-272-3900) or visit their Web site (www.alz.org) to find the location of the nearest chapter. The Alzheimer's Association can provide a wide variety of materials and information about other community resources, including telephone help lines, support groups, and living arrangement options for people with Alzheimer's disease.

Another source of information and materials about Alzheimer's disease is the Alzheimer's Disease Education and Referral Center (www.nia.nih.gov/alzheimers, 800-438-4380), a service of the National Institute on

Aging. Information on dementia and the resources available for caregivers can also be found in *The 36-Hour Day,* by Mace and Rabins (see the suggested readings).

The following Web sites also have information on dementia:

www.ninds.nih.gov (National Institute of Neurological Disorders and
   Stroke)
www.nihseniorhealth.gov (National Institutes of Health)

10

INFLUENZA AND PNEUMONIA

Influenza, usually called the flu, is a viral infection of the respiratory tract. Symptoms generally include fever, chills, dry cough, and muscle aches. For most of the 35 to 50 million Americans it strikes each year, influenza is not a serious illness. Although it is certainly unpleasant, most people are ill for only a few days and return to their regular level of activity within a couple of weeks. However, influenza is a serious health problem for high-risk groups, especially the elderly. In a typical year, 200,000 Americans are hospitalized due to influenza, and as many as 36,000 die of influenza and its complications. (In some years the figure has exceeded 40,000, and in 1918–19 more than half a million Americans died of influenza and its complications.)

Pneumonia is an infection of one or both lungs. It is caused most commonly by bacteria and, more rarely, by viruses, fungi, and other microorganisms. Pneumococcal pneumonia, a bacterial infection, is one of the most common types of pneumonia. Symptoms include fever, cough producing sputum, chest pain when inhaling, shortness of breath, headache, weakness, and fatigue. Pneumococcal pneumonia is more common in smokers, people with emphysema, and those with suppressed immune systems from HIV infection or immunosuppressive drugs (e.g., prednisone or drugs used to treat cancer or diseases like lupus or rheumatoid arthritis). Although hospitalizations and deaths due to pneumonia have decreased dramatically since the advent of antibiotics, pneumonia still results in approximately half a million hospitalizations each year and is one of the ten leading causes of death.

THE RISKS OF IGNORING INFORMATION
ON INFLUENZA AND PNEUMONIA

The greatest danger of ignoring information on influenza and pneumonia is that people in high-risk groups, especially elderly persons, will not recognize these illnesses as being serious and potentially fatal and thus will fail to take proper preventive steps. For both influenza and pneumonia, the most effective method of prevention is vaccination. Most hospitalizations and deaths resulting from influenza and pneumonia could be prevented by vaccinations. People should get influenza vaccinations on an annual basis as soon as the vaccine becomes available (typically mid-fall). Those who live with or regularly visit older adults should also be vaccinated because the vaccine prevents transmission to others. Vaccinations for pneumonia provide long-term protection and may be needed no more often than once every five to ten years. (Because recommendations vary, people should check with their physicians for more specific guidelines.)

In spite of the demonstrated effectiveness of influenza vaccinations and the fact that Medicare provides reimbursement, 30–40 percent of all Medicare beneficiaries do not get these vaccinations each year. Although the vaccination rate among African American beneficiaries has increased dramatically in recent years, non-Hispanic whites are still more likely to receive vaccinations than other racial/ethnic groups. The failure of people in high-risk groups to receive the recommended vaccination is costly in both human and economic terms. Thousands of lives and billions of dollars could be saved every year if more people would get these vaccinations.

WHAT CAN BE DONE TO PREVENT
INFLUENZA AND PNEUMONIA?

It does not appear that economic barriers are responsible for the low number of people receiving vaccinations. Vaccinations are inexpensive, reimbursed by Medicare, and relatively easy to obtain. Instead, the major barriers seem to be erroneous beliefs such as:

The vaccine can cause severe illness.
Influenza is not a serious illness.
Pneumonia can always be successfully treated with antibiotics.

People can get influenza from an influenza vaccination.
An influenza vaccination is effective for several years.
"I am not at risk."

These beliefs interfere with people's taking the necessary steps to avoid what can be serious, life-threatening illnesses. People in high-risk groups need to be given information that will encourage them to get vaccinations for influenza and pneumonia. High-risk groups that need this information are:

- People 50 years of age or older (previously this group was 65 years of age or older)
- Health care personnel
- People 18–49 years of age who have chronic medical conditions such as lung, cardiovascular, liver, kidney, or neuromuscular diseases; or metabolic disorders such as diabetes; or weakened immune systems
- People of any age who live or work with or care for members of high-risk groups and thus could easily transmit influenza

The 2007 Advisory Committee on Immunization Practices (ACIP) recommended that all adults who want to reduce their risk of becoming ill with influenza or of transmitting influenza to others should be vaccinated.

SUGGESTIONS FOR CONGREGATIONAL PROGRAMS

Make a special effort to distribute information to classes and groups that consist primarily of older adults.

Provide members of your congregation and community with information about the times and places they can receive vaccinations. This information can be obtained from your public health department or local hospitals.

Arrange to offer influenza vaccinations at your congregational facility. The public health department, local hospital, or a home health agency should be able to provide nurses and supplies. Arrange transportation to sites that provide vaccinations if you are unable to arrange for vaccinations to be given on-site.

Coordinate your congregational efforts with national public awareness campaigns. The national campaign to educate people about the benefits of influenza vaccinations usually starts in mid-October.

Use congregational bulletins and mailings to give members information about the potentially serious consequences of influenza and pneumonia and the definite benefits of vaccinations.

Develop an outreach program to provide logistical support to a health care agency to encourage vaccination among poor, underserved, and marginalized groups.

EXAMPLES OF CONGREGATIONAL PROGRAMS

An example of the impact that clergy, congregational volunteers, and health care professionals can have when they work together is an influenza vaccination program held at the San Jose Mission in Barberville, Florida. This mission, an outreach of St. Peter Catholic Church in DeLand, Florida, ministers primarily to the Hispanic population of a rural community north of DeLand. A lay health educator from St. Peter's felt that many parishioners at the San Jose Mission were likely to be unaware of the dangers of influenza and that it would be wise to offer vaccinations to all age groups in this congregation. Working closely with the county health department, she arranged to have free vaccinations offered at the mission immediately after the Sunday service. She also enlisted the assistance of the priest who encouraged everyone to be vaccinated immediately after the Sunday Mass. The response was overwhelming. Ninety parishioners were vaccinated, and many others wished to be vaccinated, but unfortunately the health department's staff had brought only ninety doses. However, pleased with the enthusiastic response of the congregation, the staff offered to return the following Sunday to offer additional vaccinations. Another ninety members were vaccinated at that time.

An example of a health care system working with faith communities to increase the number of people receiving influenza vaccinations is the program sponsored by Sacred Heart Health System in Pensacola, Florida. This program is coordinated by Cheryl Pilling, M.A., B.S.N., director of both the Faith Community Nursing Program and the Community Wellness Outreach Department. Using the Mission in Motion mobile health unit that is equipped to take preventive care (e.g., blood pressure checks, cholesterol and blood sugar screenings) to a four-county region, every fall she and other nurses arrange to offer vaccinations at several congregations. They give each congregation the option of opening the site to the general public and have found that they always do. Another important part of this program is distributing educational materials from the Centers for Disease Control and Prevention to help alert people to the risk of potentially serious complications of influenza and to help overcome some of the misconceptions about the influenza vaccine (e.g., "I'll get the flu if I get vaccinated.") that often keep people from getting vaccinated.

INFORMATION RESOURCES

Hospitals, home health agencies, and public health departments are good local resources for programs on influenza and pneumonia. In many communities these organizations will sponsor annual influenza vaccination campaigns and welcome the participation of religious congregations. The Centers for Disease Control and Prevention (www.cdc.gov/flu) is a national resource that can provide much of the information and many of the materials you will need for your programs.

The American Lung Association (www.lungusa.org, 800-LUNG-USA) also can provide information on influenza and pneumonia. Information on influenza and pneumonia can also be found at:

www.medicare.gov/health/flu.asp
www.medicare.gov/health/pneumococcal.asp

11

ADVANCE DIRECTIVES

The basis for preparing an advance directive regarding health care is the moral and legal right of every adult to accept or refuse recommended medical treatments. Colloquially, this is a direct expression of each person's fundamental right to say, "Keep your hands off me." Each person can decide what medical care to accept and what to reject. Physicians, hospitals, and nursing homes must respect the wishes of competent adults even if they disagree with certain decisions. Some people may decide that they do not want to accept a medical treatment or be on a type of life support system if they have a terminal or progressive illness and functional or cognitive disabilities.

If an injury or illness prevents a person from making decisions or communicating wishes, however, the situation may become far more complicated. Often the hardest decisions about life-sustaining or invasive treatments must be made by others, usually family members, who do not know whether their loved one would or would not want treatment. Therefore, it is advisable for adults of all ages to do some advance planning and use one or more advance directives to convey their wishes and decisions. The two most common ways for a person to provide guidance are to leave specific instructions, often called a living will, or to designate and authorize someone to make medical decisions in the event of incapacity.

A living will is a document that allows you to specify which treatments you would or would not want if you become incapacitated. The authority of living wills is limited: in most states they apply only to people who have a terminal illness or are in a persistent vegetative state (a neurologic diagnosis when an individual can breathe independently and appears to have sleep-wake cycles but has no consciousness or capability for human inter-action). For example, you can direct that you not be put on a ventilator if you are incapacitated and terminally ill or in a persistent vegetative state. If you have severe dementia and face the same decision, however, a living will would not be relevant in most states.

Because it is difficult to anticipate all the medical conditions you might encounter or all the treatments that might be available, and because living wills are so limited, it may be preferable to designate a person to make decisions on your behalf if you cannot speak for yourself. Based on an in-dividual state law or regulation, such an instrument is called a durable power of attorney for health care, a health care agent, or any of several other names. This document does not require that you be terminally ill or in a persistent vegetative state for the named individual to make medical decisions for you, only that you be incapacitated and unable to make or communicate your own decisions. Therefore, it is more broadly applicable than a living will, and the advantages of this designation were recognized by the President's Council on Bioethics in 2005.

Designating a substitute has an additional benefit. If the substitute agrees to act on your behalf, she or he must try to determine what *you* would have chosen if you could have foreseen your current situation. So the doctor would not say to her or him, "Do you think we should stop treat-ment for your mother?" Instead, the doctor should say, "What do you think your mother would tell us to do if she could be fully here with us for just a moment?" This is comforting to many adult children who do not want to feel somehow responsible for a parent's death.

Following federal regulations, hospitals and nursing homes must pro-vide patients with information about advance directives and give them an opportunity to complete these documents upon admission. Obviously, this may be a stressful time, and it is not the best time to consider such matters carefully and make important decisions. It is difficult for patients to gather all the information about the various medical circumstances they may encounter, carefully weigh their options, and then communicate their wishes to their family and physician at the time of admission. Ideally, these matters should be investigated and the documents completed at a time when a person is not so ill as to require admission to a hospital or nursing home. Later, the documents can be revised as needed.

"Do not resuscitate" orders can also be a part of advance medical planning. These orders, placed on a hospital or nursing home chart, inform the staff that the patient does not wish to undergo cardiopulmonary resuscitation if he or she experiences cardiac arrest. In some jurisdictions, individuals can keep "do not resuscitate" directives in their homes so that those responding to a 911 call for emergency care do not initiate unwanted interventions. Patients' physicians can provide them with additional information and advice about this subject.

THE RISKS OF FAILING TO USE ADVANCE DIRECTIVES

People who fail to use advance directives run the risk of receiving treatment or medical care that they would not have wanted and perhaps of being kept alive under conditions they would find unacceptable. In addition, major decisions about their medical care could be made by individuals who have different values and expectations.

The absence of advance planning can also result in painful and destructive conflicts among family members. One member of the family may feel strongly that the patient would not want to be kept on life support systems, whereas another family member may feel equally strongly that it would be wrong to withdraw the support. When there is conflict and the patient has not completed a living will or designated a substitute decision maker, the health care facility and doctor may need to choose a decision maker from a predetermined list of relatives; legal involvement becomes more likely; and the decision that is ultimately made may not reflect the patient's wishes.

An example of the challenging situations that can confront a patient and family when advance directives were not established before the end of life neared is provided by Dr. Thomas Finucane, a Johns Hopkins geriatrician who consulted with us on this chapter.

A delightful 84-year-old man with emphysema was diagnosed with incurable lung cancer. Soon thereafter he developed pneumonia and was put on a ventilator. After several days in the intensive care unit, it became clear that he could not survive without the ventilator. The difficult medical choice confronting the patient and family, as well as the medical team, was to discontinue the ventilator, allowing the man to die as comfortably as medically possible, or to continue the ventilator and allow the advancing cancer to result in death within a few months at most. The patient was thinking clearly, and we asked him which of these options he preferred. By writing on a tablet, he replied, "I don't know. Ask my wife and son."

This story exemplifies the complexity of care at the end of a life, and the realities that patients and their loved ones can confront if they have not delineated advance directives.

WHAT CAN BE DONE TO PREVENT LOSS OF CONTROL OVER MEDICAL DECISIONS?

Most people are aware of advance directives—at least the living will—and are in favor of using them. However, surveys show that few adults have formally expressed their wishes and completed the appropriate forms. One reason that people fail to complete the forms is that both physicians and patients are reluctant to broach the subject. Therefore, it is important to encourage people to discuss this matter with their physicians. They should not wait for their physicians to take the initiative.

Some people mistakenly believe that they must have an attorney prepare a living will or a durable power of attorney for health care and are reluctant to incur the costs associated with hiring one. Fortunately, establishing advance directives does not require the services of an attorney. Forms can be obtained from hospitals, home health agencies, and several national organizations. Furthermore, the forms obtained from these organizations can be modified to suit each person's wishes. Another option is for people to write their own advance directives. These are legal and acceptable directives as long as they are properly witnessed by two adults, only one of whom may be a member of the immediate family and neither of whom may be designated as the surrogate decision maker. They are, however, subject to the same restrictions as the more formal documents.

Another misconception held by some people is that they will permanently lose control of decisions about their medical care once a living will or durable power of attorney for health care has been prepared and signed. They think they are signing a document that is permanent and irrevocable. However, these documents are used only when patients are unable to communicate their wishes. Furthermore, people can change or revoke an advance directive at any time, including naming another individual to hold a durable power of attorney for health care. Finally, wishes can change as the end of life approaches, and until one is confronted by the realities of an illness, it is not always possible to accurately predict what you will want. Thus, beginning to think and talk through these matters when well can ease the discussions later.

People need to be encouraged to discuss their wishes and feelings about end-of-life matters with family members or other designated decision makers. These individuals need to know that the documents exist and that they were executed after careful consideration of the medical circumstances and options. A statement or declaration of personal values completed by the patient can be helpful to family members who need to understand the patient's wishes and decisions. Additionally, a statement of values can serve as a helpful guide for a person who has the durable power of attorney for health care.

SUGGESTIONS FOR CONGREGATIONAL PROGRAMS

Use congregational bulletins and mailings to provide members of your congregation with information about advance directives. Information and sample forms can be obtained from hospitals and home health agencies.

Sponsor a program on advance directives. A physician, nurse, or social worker can provide information about medical circumstances patients might encounter and decisions they might face. An attorney can offer information on required formalities in your state and advise how to personalize these documents.

Sponsor a program on ethical decision making. This could be led by the clergy and could include examples of statements or declarations of values.

Arrange for members of your congregation to videotape their wishes and instructions on end-of-life matters. This videotape could then be used to supplement written documents if the situation arises.

EXAMPLES OF CONGREGATIONAL PROGRAMS

During a Shabbat service at Temple Beth El in Ormond Beach, Florida, Rabbi Altman asked the members to stay after the service to hear brief presentations on advance directives by Dr. Alvin Smith, a well-known oncologist (who was not a member of the congregation) and Marshall Barkin, an attorney (who was a member). Dr. Smith offered several examples of situations in which patients with terminal illnesses who had lost their ability to communicate with others were forced to receive medical treatment they probably did not want. However, because they had not prepared advance directives expressing their wishes, the doctor and hospital were forced to continue the treatment. He strongly urged members of the congregation to avoid these situations by completing a living will and designating a trusted individual as their surrogate decision maker. Mr. Barkin, the attorney, provided additional information about these documents and further encouraged members to use them. Rabbi Altman then reinforced their advice by also recommending that members take these measures to ensure that their wishes about end-of-life care would be honored.

Leslie Piet, a registered nurse in Bel Air, Maryland, who works with people who have cancer and serves on the board of Aging with Dignity, adopted a different approach to spreading the word about advance directives—she hosted a "living wills party" at her house. Thirty members of her church gathered at her home one evening. They were first given copies of Five Wishes, a widely used living will form and then shown a 25-minute videotape produced by Aging with Dignity that describes the Five Wishes form and how to use it. Following this, Leslie facilitated a discussion about advance directives and answered their questions. Several people then completed their forms, while others said they wanted to take the forms home to discuss their concerns and wishes with their families. One of the church members at this party, an 87-year-old woman who was going in for a total hip replacement, was particularly insistent about completing her form. Everyone who attended seemed pleased to learn about advance directives and to have an opportunity to discuss the topic with others. Soon word of this gathering spread, and Leslie received several requests to hold another one, which she did. Her church now keeps copies of Five Wishes on hand for anyone who asks to have one. Leslie's idea of having a "living wills party" or an "advance directives party" caught the attention of a reporter for *USA Today* who, in an article on living wills (April 27, 2005), featured her party along with advice for others interested in sponsoring similar events.

INFORMATION RESOURCES

Hospitals and home health agencies can provide copies of advance directives, and many will arrange for knowledgeable speakers to give presentations to community groups. Many attorneys will also volunteer their time to speak to groups about advance directives.

Several national organizations provide information and materials on advance directives. Caring Connections (www.caringinfo.org), a program of the National Hospice and Palliative Care Organization, provides advice on preparing for end-of-life care and also free downloadable advance directives and instructions for each state. The American Bar Association's Commission on Law and Aging offers on its Web site (www.abanet.org/aging/toolkit/home.html) a "Tool Kit for Health Care Advance Planning." The materials in this tool kit can help people identify some of the key issues they should consider as they prepare advance directives. Another resource is Aging with Dignity (www.agingwithdignity.org). This organization provides, at a nominal charge, copies of "Five Wishes," a living will that addresses in easy-to-understand language the medical, personal, emotional, and spiritual needs of a seriously ill person. This document is available in English and 20 other languages, including Arabic, French, Haitian Creole, Hindi, Korean, Spanish, and Vietnamese. A video, *Five Wishes,* can also be obtained through Aging with Dignity.

12

COMMUNICATING WITH
HEALTH CARE PROVIDERS

Many patients have had the experience of coming out of a meeting with their physician feeling more confused than when they went in. It is not unusual for patients to report that they do not completely understand their illness or what they should do to manage their condition more effectively, even though they have had several meetings with their doctor. Many factors can contribute to this confusion and uncertainty. Some of the obstacles patients frequently mention include:

Medical terminology: "My doctor acted like I should understand the terminology he was using. I would have felt stupid telling him I didn't."

Doctor's schedule: "The doctor seemed too busy to discuss all of my concerns. She looked rushed, and there were so many other patients in her waiting room."

Patient's anxiety: "I was so nervous about my situation that I forgot to tell him something important."

Patient's attitude: "I find it difficult to question or be assertive with my doctor. It's easier to just listen quietly."

Doctor's interview style: "My doctor's questions led me away from some of the things I had intended to discuss. I never got back to several of my concerns."

Information overload: "There was just too much information. I was overwhelmed."

Problems with memory: "I understood what she said, but by the time I got home, I had forgotten most of it."

These and other problems can interfere with the exchange of clear, accurate information between a patient and his or her doctor. Without good two-way communication, the medical encounter cannot reach its full potential and may, in some cases, prove ineffective or even counterproductive. Physicians need accurate information from patients if they are to arrive at a correct diagnosis and formulate an effective treatment plan, and patients need information about their condition and recommended treatment that is clear, relevant, and useful if the treatment plan is to be implemented correctly and then maintained.

Although many factors can contribute to the problem of poor communication between patients and physicians, patients can use a few key strategies to overcome these obstacles, and the benefits of adopting these strategies are well established. Patients who take the initiative to improve communication with their physicians receive more factual information from their physicians, are more likely to follow through with treatment recommendations, and report greater satisfaction with the care they are receiving.

An important point for patients to remember as they prepare for medical visits is that most significant issues can be covered during a meeting with a physician if the information is well organized and presented in a direct, clear manner. Physicians are trained to take in and process large amounts of information in a relatively brief period of time. The key to a successful meeting with a physician is for the patient to have a well-organized, carefully prepared outline that covers all the important items he or she wishes to discuss.

We have written a brief guide, Making the Most of Your Medical Visit, that individuals can use as they prepare for their medical visits and during their meetings with physicians. It also has advice and suggestions that address some of the concerns or questions that often emerge after patients have left their physician's office. This guide can be copied and distributed to interested persons. It is also available in PDF format on the Web site of the O'Neill Foundation for Community Health (www.oneillcommunityhealth .org) and can be downloaded and copied.

MAKING THE MOST OF YOUR MEDICAL VISIT
Preparing for Your Medical Visit

One of the best ways to demonstrate to your physician that you want to be an active and informed participant in your health care is taking with you to your appointment some basic information about your medical situation and a list of three or four questions that you would like answered. Be sure to let your doctor know at the beginning of the visit that you have this information and several questions. This will show that you have given thought to the medical issues of greatest concern to you and that you want to make good use of your time together. It is a good idea to write your questions on a card or sheet of paper in case your doctor's answer to one of your questions shifts your attention away from your other concerns.

To answer your questions, arrive at a correct diagnosis, and formulate an effective treatment plan, your physician will need certain information from you. Below are a number of questions that can help you organize this information and prepare for your appointment.

What is your primary concern? What problem or problems do you want your physician to address? For example, is your primary objective to have your condition diagnosed and treated as aggressively as possible or to find a treatment that minimizes pain and allows you to continue with activities you enjoy? Sometimes physicians are so focused on identifying and treating the underlying disease that they do not give enough attention to certain aspects of the disease or treatments that are of concern to patients.

What symptoms are you experiencing? Be as specific as possible. When did they begin? If they are not constant, then at what times or in what situations do they occur? What makes them improve or become worse? Have you ever had these symptoms before? If so, how long ago and how were they treated? How is this illness affecting your day-to-day life?

What is your understanding of the problem? Perhaps you have discussed your problem with a friend or consulted a Web site or medical book. (Many of the health-related Web sites are excellent, but there are also many that are not reliable. Chapter 18 lists some of the most reliable Web sites.) If you have some ideas about what you are experiencing or what has caused the problem, be prepared to share these with your physician.

What remedies have you already tried? Have you taken any over-the-counter medications? Have you changed your diet or modified any of your habits in an attempt to address the problem? If so, did your efforts help?

Are you being treated for any other problems by another physician or health care professional? If so, who are you seeing and for what problem(s)?

What medications, including nonprescription medications and nutritional supplements, are you currently taking? Often the best way to provide this information for your physician is to carry all your medications with you to your appointment.

Have there been any significant changes in your life since your last appointment (e.g., illness or death of a loved one, difficulties in relationships with family or friends, new living arrangements, change in financial status, new responsibilities at home or at work, change in your ability to handle household matters)?

How have you been feeling emotionally lately? Have you felt anxious or depressed about your health or anything else going on in your life?

Are there any potential obstacles to the treatment or additional diagnostic tests your physician might recommend (e.g., financial limitations, family or work responsibilities)?

Have you completed any advance directives (e.g., a living will, durable power of attorney for health care)? If so, be sure to take copies with you and ask your physician to add them to your chart. If not, then consider discussing these with your physician.

One more step you should seriously consider as you prepare for your visit to your physician is to ask a family member or friend to accompany you. If you think it might be difficult for you to present all the information that needs to be presented or to ask important questions or to remember what your doctor is recommending, then ask someone to go with you to your appointment.

Meeting with Your Doctor

Remember to take your basic medical information and your questions with you along with paper and pen to record the information and recommendations your physician will be giving you. Also carry all your medications, both prescription and nonprescription, or at least a detailed list of these medications. If you are having someone accompany you, be sure to clarify what role you want him or her to play during your visit.

If a nurse or medical assistant takes your blood pressure before you see the physician, ask for the results and record these. Later, during your examination, ask your doctor what he or she thinks about your blood pressure.

When your physician arrives and begins questioning you, start off by explaining your primary reason for the visit, being as specific as you can about your symptoms, concerns, and hopes. Also mention that you have several questions you need to ask before you leave.

When sharing information about your symptoms and what you believe they may indicate, be as specific, complete, and organized as possible. Exactly what are you experiencing now and how does that differ from what you normally experience? If some of your symptoms suggest to you a certain diagnosis, perhaps based on what someone else told you or what you read on a Web site or in a medical book, then report those symptoms and ask if they might be an indication of a particular condition. For example, if you have had difficulty sleeping, have lost weight, and no longer enjoy activities you previously found pleasurable, and have read that these might be an indication of depression, share this information and ask if this means you might be depressed. This will enable your physician to ask the relevant questions and determine if that is the correct diagnosis.

If you believe that your medical problem might be related to stress you are experiencing or something you have done or some aspect of your lifestyle, share this with your physician. If you are concerned that this information would prove embarrassing if family members or friends were to learn about it, ask your physician to clarify exactly how he or she handles information that you want to be kept in confidence. (Also, remember that federal laws enacted in recent years strictly limit what information health care practitioners can share with or tell others—even a spouse—without a patient's express written approval.)

If your physician does not ask if you are seeing any other health professionals or receiving treatment for other problems, go ahead and volunteer this information. Be sure to include treatments that may not be strictly medical (e.g., acupuncture, nutritional or herbal supplements, chiropractic care, homeopathy). Also, let your doctor know about the medications, prescription and nonprescription, that you are taking.

As your doctor conducts a physical examination, do not be reluctant to ask if he or she has found anything of importance. Did your heart sound okay? What about your lungs? If he or she seems to spend more time on one part of the examination, ask why? This would also be a good time to inquire about your blood pressure.

Following the physical examination and your report of your symptoms, concerns, medications, and other medical problems for which you are being treated, your physician may be able to give you a diagnosis. This should be in terms that you understand. If you do not understand the terminology used, do not hesitate to speak up and ask for clarification. In fact, even if you are relatively confident that you understand the diagnosis, it is a good idea to repeat it and to put into your own words your understanding of the condition. We recommend that you or the person who has accompanied you to your appointment write down the diagnosis and explanation and then ask the doctor to read over what has been written to be sure that it is correct.

If for some reason you do not believe that the diagnosis you have been given is correct or that the recommended treatment will be effective, voice your doubts to your physician and explain why you disagree. It is far better to politely and respectfully express your doubts during the appointment than to keep your thoughts to yourself and then, once you leave your appointment, disregard your physician's opinion and recommendations.

It is generally advisable to ask what has caused this condition or what factors have contributed to its development. For many chronic conditions, there is more than one contributing factor, so it may be difficult for your physician to give a definitive answer to this question, but he or she should be able to provide you a general explanation. Here again, we recommend that you repeat and then write down the information about contributing factors.

Once the diagnosis has been determined and contributing factors discussed, your physician will offer treatment recommendations. Often this will include a prescription for one or more medications. It is important that you understand exactly what is being prescribed and why it is being prescribed. Estimates are that as many as 50 percent or more of patients do not take their medications appropriately. Frequently this is because of a breakdown in communication between physician and patient.

If your physician does not volunteer enough information about the medication, you need to ask a number of questions. Exactly what are the expected benefits of the medication? How long will it take for you to notice the benefits? How should it be taken? Is any other medication you are taking likely to interfere with this one, or is this medication likely to interfere with any of your other medications? Is this a medication that will need to be taken only for a limited period of time or is it likely that you will need to remain on it indefinitely? Is it possible that you will experience some side effects? If so, what should you do? Be sure to write down the answers to these questions and review your notes with your physician before you leave.

If there is any reason why you might not be able to take the medication you have been prescribed, do not hesitate to mention this to your physician. Doctors understand and appreciate the fact that the latest and best medication for a particular medical condition is of no value if it is not taken as prescribed. If the cost of the medication will prevent you from obtaining it, explain this to your physician. Doctors often can prescribe a less expensive alternative that has similar benefits. If your work schedule or other aspects of your life make it unlikely that you will be able to take the medication at the times prescribed, ask your physician if there is a similar medication that would be more compatible with your daily routine.

It is possible your physician will determine that what are generally referred to as lifestyle factors are contributing to your condition and that these need to be modified. This recommendation often presents at least two challenges for patients. First, many patients do not think of a change in physical activity or diet as a *medical* treatment. To them, this type of recommendation does not seem to be as important as a recommendation to take a prescribed medication. Therefore, it is important that you have a clear understanding of the connection between these lifestyle factors and your condition. How will a change in your behavior affect your medical condition? What will happen if you do not make the recommended changes?

Second, even when patients understand the connection between certain lifestyle factors and their condition, it can be difficult to modify habits that are deeply ingrained and often highly pleasurable. Patients need to recognize this and ask for help implementing and maintaining the recommended changes. For some problems (e.g., smoking), your physician may be able to prescribe medication that will help. If the problem with the recommended modification (e.g., adopting a low-fat diet) is that family members are unlikely to cooperate and support your efforts to change, ask if your physician would be willing to meet with them to explain the importance of these recommendations. If you believe it would be easier for you to make the recommended changes if you could be around others who were working toward a similar goal, ask your physician if he or she knows of any community groups or programs that are focused on the same problem (e.g., weight reduction).

Once you are clear about the diagnosis, contributing factors, and treatment recommendations (remember to ask questions if you are unclear about any of these matters), share with your physician your reaction to this information. Do you feel better now that you know the diagnosis and how your condition is to be treated? Are you confident that you will be able to follow the treatment recommendations? How has this information affected you emotionally? Has any of this information frightened you or discouraged you? Do you fear that your illness or the treatments are going to limit your ability to work or carry on other activities you value? If you find that you are pessimistic about your ability to carry out the treatment recommendation or feel overwhelmed emotionally by what you have heard, ask your physician for suggestions about a support group or a mental health professional who could help you.

For certain illnesses, you may want to address other issues during a visit with your doctor. If you believe that your illness is likely to progress, even with the recommended treatment, you may want to ask about the long-term course of your illness and the implications for your living arrangements. Would it be advisable for you to make some modifications in your house or apartment (e.g., grab rails, ramps)? Should you or family members begin looking for new living arrangements (e.g., an assisted living facility, a continuing care retirement community)? Will you need to consider a hospice program at some point? You also may want to get advice about what you should consider as you prepare or update advance directives.

As your visit draws to an end, be sure that you have asked all of your questions and that you understand your doctor's answers. You should have a clear understanding of your diagnosis, likely contributing factors, and treatment recommendations. If you feel it would be helpful to learn more about your illness or treatment, ask your physician if there are printed materials or if there is a reliable book or Web site you could read for more information. Finally, be certain that you know when you are to return for a subsequent appointment or when and where you need to go for additional tests.

Follow-up

The visit with your physician is an essential part of good medical care. However, for most chronic conditions, what takes place at home is just as important as what takes place at your doctor's office or the hospital. In fact, most of the recommended care will take place at home. For example, the medications prescribed by your doctor will be of little benefit if they are not taken correctly, and sound advice about lifestyle modifications is of no value if it is not followed. Therefore, it is important for you to take the steps needed to implement treatment recommendations and to do so as soon as you can after visiting your doctor.

It is not uncommon for questions about your illness and/or the treatment recommendations to arise after you have left the doctor's office. You may find that the medication you were prescribed does not seem to be having the beneficial effects you were expecting or that it is producing some unpleasant side effects. Or perhaps you are no longer experiencing the symptoms that prompted your medical visit and thus are not certain that you need to continue taking your medication. Any questions about whether or not to continue taking a medication should be made in consultation with your physician. You should, at a minimum, call your doctor's office and express your concerns. If you have discovered that the medication you have been prescribed is too expensive or not on the list of medications covered by your insurance policy, you may want to ask your pharmacist about alternatives and request that he or she contact your physician to see if the prescription can be changed.

Sometimes an illness is unusual or rare and getting the opinion of another physician or specialist is appropriate. You may not necessarily understand or know when this is the case, but asking your physician whether or not a consultation from another specialist is worthwhile is always a reasonable thing to do. When exceptionally rare or life-threatening conditions are diagnosed, or if a major operation is recommended, you may be comforted by getting a second opinion from another physician concerning the recommended course of treatment. Often, it is advisable to turn to a regional or national academic medical center in these cases. To prepare for such a visit, you should gather and send all appropriate medical records to the expert physician being consulted so that she or he is prepared to meet with you knowing as much information as possible about your condition and the concerns you want to be addressed (e.g., recommendations regarding treatment, need for further testing, consideration of other approaches to diagnosis and treatment).

If blood work or other tests were conducted during or shortly after your medical visit, take the initiative to check back with your doctor's office to get the results and to see if you need to return for another appointment or make any changes in your treatment. Given the complexity of modern medicine, test results can return to a physician's office within hours of your visit (e.g., routine blood work) or take days or even weeks for final results to be released. Particularly for radiology (e.g., X-rays, mammograms, MRIs) or pathology (e.g., skin biopsies), test results and receipt of reports can be delayed. Therefore, it is important for you to track and ensure that your doctor receives the final report and that any critical information is shared with you.

Good communication between patients and doctors is essential to good medical care, and you can do your part by following these three basic recommendations:

- Be prepared for your visit with your doctor. Organize key information about your medical situation and prepare several questions you would like answered.
- Be active during your appointment. Ask questions and do not hesitate to request clarification if you do not understand your doctor's answers.
- Follow through on your doctor's recommendations. If there is a reason you cannot, get back in touch with your doctor to explore other alternatives.

THE PATIENT ADVOCATE OR HEALTH PARTNER

One of the recommendations in the guide, Making the Most of Your Medical Visit, is for people to ask a family member or friend to accompany them to their appointments. This can be especially important for those who have multiple chronic conditions and thus require a variety of medications or treatments. Unfortunately, some individuals do not have a family member or friend who is able to serve in this capacity. One way religious congregations can assist these individuals is to recruit and prepare volunteers to fill this role. Working closely with health care professionals and religious leaders, we have prepared a brief guide for members of congregations who are interested in serving as patient advocates or health partners, helping patients prepare for medical visits, and then accompanying them to their appointments. This guide, Serving as a Patient Advocate, can be copied and used for training and guidance. It is also available in PDF format on the Web site of the O'Neill Foundation for Community Health (www .oneillcommunityhealth.org) and can be downloaded and copied. The guide can be supplemented with the advice of an experienced physician or nurse familiar with the local medical community and health care system.

SERVING AS A PATIENT ADVOCATE OR HEALTH PARTNER

The goal of a patient advocate program is to train people to work on a one-to-one basis with older adults and others who need assistance managing chronic illnesses and medical conditions. The primary responsibility of patient advocates is to serve as an extra pair of eyes and ears when patients are interacting with their physicians, facilitating the flow of information between patients and physicians. Once medical information has been exchanged, patients often need assistance in following their physician's recommendations. For example, patients often find it difficult to remember follow-up appointments or to consistently comply with their doctor's recommendations about medications. Patient advocates can help patients organize their schedules and medicines and then provide further assistance by telephone or brief visits. Also, they can discuss with patients steps to prevent additional medical problems (e.g., injuries resulting from falls) and how to maintain control over decisions about their medical care if they become incapacitated (e.g., use of advance directives). Patient advocates can provide emotional support and reassurance for patients. However, they should not be expected to provide any financial support, nor are they to receive any financial benefits.

Although the time demands on patient advocates do not have to be great and the training required is not extensive, several special qualities are necessary to serve in this capacity. First, you must be willing to listen to and talk about difficult issues. Some of the things you may hear about and discuss with patients and physicians may not be pleasant, yet these matters must be dealt with openly and professionally to facilitate the best possible care for the patient. Furthermore, patient advocates often are entrusted with sensitive information that must be treated with *absolute confidentiality*. You must understand and accept this responsibility. The information you hear cannot be shared with anyone other than the patient unless you are clearly instructed to do so by the patient.

Second, you must be able to earn the trust of both patients and medical professionals. Although we can provide individuals with the knowledge and skills to serve as patient advocates, your effectiveness will be greatly limited if you do not have the trust and respect of patients and health care providers.

Third, you must be able to respect not only the patient's privacy but also his or her wishes. You may encounter situations in which the wishes or values of the patient conflict with your own. In these situations, you must be willing to set aside your own feelings and act on behalf of the patient. It is your responsibility to act as the agent or representative of the patient.

It is also important that you not bring your own personal agendas regarding medical care into your work. The role of the patient advocate is to serve as a facilitator, not as an adversary of physicians, nurses, or hospitals. Although you may need to be assertive and persistent in some of your efforts, you still need to feel comfortable about working within the health care system.

You will need to establish good working relationships with the patients you are assisting. This is usually a two-step process: The first step is developing rapport with the patient; the second step is clarifying your role as a patient advocate.

As a patient advocate, the best way to begin a relationship with a patient is to say a few things about yourself (e.g., your previous work experience or some of your current activities). Although you should disclose enough information about yourself so that the patient feels comfortable with you, do not go into too much detail. Keep the focus on the patient and his or her needs. As you talk with the patient, try to create a relaxed atmosphere. Let the patient see that you are comfortable talking about health matters and personal concerns.

As you develop rapport with the person you will be assisting, suggest that it would be helpful for you to explain specifically what you will be capable of doing as a patient advocate. Let the patient know how you envision your role.

One of the first matters you need to address is the issue of confidentiality. Many people we talked to about patient advocate programs expressed the concern that some of their medical problems might be discussed with acquaintances in their congregation or community. Even though a patient advocate might have good intentions about sharing information (e.g., encouraging others to provide assistance), such disclosures can undermine, and even destroy, the relationship between the patient and the patient advocate. Therefore, it is imperative that you treat all information as absolutely confidential. Only if the patient clearly gives you permission to share personal and medical information should you do so. You should take the initiative in discussing this issue because some patients may be reluctant to say anything about it even if they have concerns.

It is also important for you to clarify your limitations. You should be certain that the patient realizes that you are not a medical expert. You should not be expected to be the direct source of information or advice about medical matters. Instead, your role is to help the patient obtain the necessary information from physicians and other appropriate sources.

In addition, you need to clarify financial matters. It is not the role of a patient advocate to provide financial support for the patient. If the patient has financial problems that interfere with his or her ability to obtain recommended treatment, you may help him or her bring this to the attention of the physician, hospital social worker, or an appropriate social service agency, but you should not be expected to provide or find sources of money yourself.

Another financial matter to be addressed is the issue of a patient advocate receiving money or gifts for his or her efforts. This may be an unspoken concern of the patient's family members who are not close enough to monitor your activities. They may fear that you will obtain control over the patient's bank account and misuse the money. It is best to address this fear by suggesting that the patient contact relatives and explain your role as a patient advocate.

After you feel you have established rapport with the patient and given him or her enough information about your background, your interest in the program, and what can be expected of you, you are ready to begin gathering information about the patient's medical concerns and any related matters. The questions presented in Making the Most of Your Medical Visit can serve as a guide. A patient check sheet (see appendix C) and a patient information sheet (see appendix D) can be used in preparation for the meeting with the doctor.

The patient check sheet (appendix C) can guide you as you talk with the patient. In most cases, this form does not need to be taken to each appointment. The information you gather as you complete this form can be concisely summarized and transferred to the patient information sheet. However, as you fill out the patient check sheet, if you discover that there have been several significant changes in the patient's life since his or her last doctor's visit, it may be best to take this form with you.

The patient information sheet (appendix D) is designed to be completed before the appointment and taken to the meeting with the doctor. This sheet can help you organize the information the physician needs and establish a prioritized problem list.

As you talk with the patient, do not hesitate to speak up if you are confused by something the patient has said. If you do not understand a term or are uncertain about what the patient means, tell him or her that you are confused. This will let the patient know that you are genuinely interested in understanding what he or she is saying.

If the patient expresses a sense of loss or emotional pain related to his or her illness, do not try to provide immediate relief or reassurance. Give the patient ample opportunity to talk about fears or losses. The danger of offering reassurance too quickly is that the patient may think that you do not understand his or her feelings or do not even wish to.

Do not rush to fill silent periods in your conversations. Give the patient time to think and respond. Silent periods can be valuable to both of you. He or she may need time to reflect on some issues you have raised, and you can use these periods both to review what has been discussed thus far and to observe the patient's nonverbal behavior. If you think the patient's eyes or facial expression reveals a certain emotion, share your observations. For example, if you think you detect fear, gently ask if this is what he or she is experiencing.

Finally, try not to be surprised or shocked by the unexpected. You may assume that the patient feels a certain way because that is how you would feel or because you know how other people have reacted under similar circumstances. Although it is helpful to draw on your own experiences or those of others, recognize that not everyone reacts in the same manner.

When you and the patient have finished preparing for the visit to the doctor, you need to discuss what your role will be at the doctor's office or hospital. Some patients will want you to accompany them into their meeting with the doctor to assist them in explaining their concerns and help them record the doctor's explanations and recommendations. In these situations, it is advisable for you or the patient to explain to the doctor who you are and why you are there. Also mention that you will excuse yourself during the physical examination but that you would like to be brought back into the meeting so that you can hear the doctor's recommendations.

A form entitled "Summary Form for Physician Visit" (see appendix E) can be used for recording the doctor's explanations and recommendations. Because the goal of recording the doctor's recommendations is to facilitate the accurate and complete exchange of information, it is important that you ask the physician to review and confirm what you have written down. Have the doctor initial the form on the line at the bottom.

Another way you can assist the patient is to encourage him or her to be assertive in expressing concerns to the doctor. Many patients find it difficult to be assertive with their physicians. Some feel that it is disrespectful to question the doctor's opinions and recommendations or to offer information that is not specifically requested. Instead, these patients adopt a passive role, allowing their doctor to ask all the questions and set the direction for discussion. They see their doctor as the source of all knowledge and expertise. Other patients are skeptical of their doctor's advice, but they do not share their feelings directly with the doctor. They keep their opinions to themselves during their appointment, but once they leave, they disregard the doctor's recommendations.

Although it may seem obvious that patients need to express themselves while meeting with their physicians, it is not easy for some people to be assertive, especially with authority figures who seem to be so knowledgeable. It is important for patients to realize that they also possess valuable expertise when the subject is their own health. They need to remember that they have important information that needs to be communicated to their physician and that good, comprehensive care can be provided only when they share this information. Gentle reminders from you can help patients become more confident and assertive.

As a patient advocate, you can play a valuable role in helping patients benefit from the medications that have been prescribed. In fact, physicians consider this one of the most important roles for patient advocates. Here are several suggestions you can follow to improve patient compliance with taking medications:

- Ask the patient, "Do you understand why your physician has prescribed the medication?" The patient should know what the medication is for, how to take it, and what to expect. If the patient does not understand why the medication was prescribed, encourage him or her to check with the physician.
- Write down the information and instructions provided by the patient's physician. Take notes while you are in the doctor's office. Space is provided on the "Summary Form for Physician Visit" (see appendix E).
- Encourage the patient to ask his or her primary care physician to review all the patient's medications. Suggest that the patient take all his or her medications, or at least a list of the medications, to the doctor's appointment. Include over-the-counter (nonprescription) drugs and nutritional and herbal supplements.
- Advise the patient to report any unexpected or unpleasant side effects to the doctor.
- Suggest that the patient use one pharmacist or pharmacy for all his or her medications and encourage the patient to accept medication counseling when it is offered by the pharmacist.
- Advise the patient to ask his or her pharmacist to contact the doctor when a medication is too expensive. A less expensive alternative may be available.
- Encourage the patient to use medication organizers or pillboxes.
- Help the patient keep a record of his or her medications. The record should include information about the medication, what it is for, color and shape, the time it is to be taken, any concerns or problems related to it, and how regularly the patient takes it as prescribed. Appendix F provides a sample medication record.

Most important, encourage the patient to communicate openly with his or her physician about medications. The patient should not hesitate to ask questions or report difficulties with the medication.

SUGGESTIONS FOR CONGREGATIONAL PROGRAMS

Invite a local physician who is known as a good communicator to speak on the topic of doctor-patient communication and how patients can handle difficult issues with their physicians.

Sponsor a program on how to find reliable medical information on the Internet. If your hospital has a medical library, one of the librarians could serve as your speaker.

Invite a representative from your hospital to talk about medical tests commonly ordered by physicians.

Invite a primary care physician to discuss how he or she conducts physical examinations.

Invite a physician or nurse to lead a program on medical terminology commonly used with patients.

Sponsor a training program for members interested in learning how to become a patient advocate. This could be led by a physician or nurse.

EXAMPLE OF A CONGREGATIONAL PROGRAM

Heart and Soul Food Pantry/Dining Room, located in Niagara Falls, New York, is an outstanding example of how to provide a special ministry outside the doors of the church and how to provide assistance to individuals who may have difficulty communicating with health professionals. Founded in 1981, its basic mission is to "feed those in need and provide opportunities to improve quality of life." In 2002, Mount St. Mary's Hospital and Health Care Center, a member of Ascension Health, became involved when the hospital was approached by two benefactors of Heart and Soul who were interested in having health care services provided at the soup kitchen site. Surveys and interviews indicated that an on-site health clinic was not the answer. Rather, helping guests gain access to available services, especially primary care, was the greatest need. The decision was made to place the hospital's parish nurse coordinator, Barbara Malinowski, M.S.N., R.N., at Heart and Soul to set up and coordinate a health ministry similar to those in congregations. This program would fit well into the "Ascension Call to Action: Health care that works, health care that is safe, and health care that leaves no one behind."

What began as a simple blood pressure screening program soon expanded into a program that not only provides access to health care but is mindful of the spiritual care of the clients served. The problems of the clients are often complex, and compliance with treatment recommendations is a major problem. When we think of clients who are noncompliant, we often assume that they are irresponsible, but for the clients of Heart and Soul, the failure to comply is most often the result of having no transportation, no telephone to confirm or be reminded about appointments, no health insurance, and most of all, little understanding of instructions.

The staff of the health ministry program addresses the issue of noncompliance by helping clients prepare for their medical appointments and, if necessary, accompanying them. In addition, treatment recommendations are reviewed with the clients to be sure they understand what they need to do.

An illustration of how the program provides assistance to their clients with medical needs is found in the story of Walter, which began when he stopped a parish nurse one day and told her that he wasn't feeling well—a little tired, no energy, and short of breath. In further discussion, he revealed that six years earlier he had had two stents inserted for "some type of heart blockage." He had stopped taking his medication approximately a year ago, had not had any medical follow-up, and currently had no health insurance. Fearing that Walter was in congestive heart failure, the nurse made a call to the Neighborhood Health Center, an outpatient clinic operated by Mount St. Mary's Hospital. An appointment was made that resulted in a referral to a cardiologist, where it was found that he needed bypass surgery. Because there were no family members available to assist, staff from the Health Ministry Program accompanied him to his preoperative evaluation and stayed with him on the day of surgery. The staff visited him daily at the hospital, and after he was discharged accompanied him to his post-op visit with the surgeon and follow-up visits with his cardiologist and primary care physician. Before each visit, they helped him prepare a list of questions to take with him to the doctor's appointment.

As a result of this assistance, Walter has followed his activity schedule and attended his cardiac rehabilitation classes. He has a fairly good understanding of his condition (even though he is not happy about his restrictions), and his recovery process has been steady. This would not have been the case if he had not had people to assist him in the process.

INFORMATION RESOURCES

A helpful booklet, "Talking with Your Doctor: A Guide for Older People," can be ordered or downloaded from the National Institute on Aging Web site (www.niapublications.org/pubs/talking/index.asp).

13

MODIFYING COMMON
RISK FACTORS

There are a number of risk factors for most major chronic diseases, some of which are beyond our control (e.g., age, gender, family history). But there are other risk factors, generally referred to as lifestyle factors, over which we can exert considerable influence. In this chapter we discuss four of these factors—stress, inadequate physical activity, excess weight, and smoking—and offer strategies for modifying them. For each lifestyle factor, we have written brief guides that can be copied and handed out to individuals interested in modifying that factor. These guides are also available in PDF format on the Web site of the O'Neill Foundation for Community Health (www.oneillcommunityhealth.org) and can be downloaded and copied. Each guide is followed by suggestions for congregational programs and information about additional resources.

A BRIEF GUIDE TO STRESS MANAGEMENT

Stress is an inevitable part of life, but when it is prolonged or excessive, it can adversely affect our health. For example, it can impair immune system functioning or trigger the release of hormones that speed up heart rate and raise blood pressure. But stress also can increase our risk of illness or exacerbate existing illnesses by making it more difficult for us to maintain health-enhancing behavior patterns (e.g., regular exercise, healthy diet). Therefore, it is important for us to learn how to manage stress effectively.

The first step in managing stress is to identify what is causing it. Although this might appear to be a simple assignment—you may quickly point to new responsibilities at work or a crisis within the family (or both)—it is not always clear exactly why the situation is stressful or what elements of the situation make it so. Two people can face the same challenging situation and yet differ dramatically in their reactions. Often it is helpful to keep a journal in which you record not only the various tasks you have each day but also your thoughts about these tasks and your ability to handle them. Exactly what did you do? Who else was involved? What was said? How did you feel about what you did? It is also a good idea to keep track of the activities that you enjoyed each day and the times you were able to break free of the stressful situation and relax.

The next step is to carefully analyze your daily activities and thoughts. Which task or tasks caused the most stress? Was there one particular responsibility you found stressful, or was the stress you experienced the result of having to handle too many responsibilities? Did the people with whom you interacted add to or reduce the stress? What did you say to yourself about how you handled your responsibilities? Did you feel you did a good job? Was the task as difficult or overwhelming as you had anticipated? How much time did you have to do some of the things you enjoy? What situations or activities did you find relaxing or renewing?

Your next step depends on what you discovered through your analysis of your daily activities. Below are some typical causes of stress and strategies for addressing each.

"I have too many responsibilities." This is a common problem, and there are different approaches to managing this source of stress. First, prioritize your various responsibilities or tasks, and then ask yourself several questions: Which are the essential tasks—the ones you absolutely have to continue? Are there any that you can set aside or ask someone else to take over? Frequently we are reluctant to step back from responsibilities or hand them off to others, but there may come a time when you need to do this in order to carry out your most important responsibilities and, at the same time, maintain your own health.

Improving your time management skills also may help. Often, when new responsibilities have been added, a person's life becomes disorganized. Whereas previously you were able to handle all your responsibilities without giving much thought to your schedule or relying on a planner, you now find that everything seems to be in disarray. It can be helpful to set aside enough time to list each day's responsibilities, establish priorities, and create a realistic plan for handling these responsibilities. Many find that using a daily or weekly planner is helpful. And when you are filling in your planner, be sure to schedule some time for yourself! Treat this time, even if it is only a few minutes, as a high priority item, essential to maintaining the good health you need to carry out your responsibilities.

"Other people are expecting too much of me," or *"I'm not getting the help that I need."* If your analysis has revealed that other people seem to have unrealistic expectations of you, or if you have found that individuals who could be assisting you are not doing so, then it may be helpful to work on improving your communication skills. This is not to say that you have had poor communication skills, but new circumstances may call for a change in your approach.

Chances are that at least some of the people with whom you interact are not aware that you are feeling overwhelmed by your responsibilities. They may not know about all of your various duties, or you may give the appearance that everything is under control and that you do not need any help. The only way these individuals are going to come to your aid is if you take the initiative to say in an assertive manner what you are feeling about your situation and your needs. But before you do this, it is important to understand what assertive communication is and is not. The purpose of assertive communication is to clearly express your feelings and needs—not to attack or criticize someone else.

The best way to handle assertive communication, especially during a crisis or period of great stress, is to identify exactly what you need to say, plan how to say it, and even rehearse it a few times. And remember, the goal is to communicate what you need, not to criticize others. For example, a simple statement, "I am feeling overwhelmed and really need some help," is more effective than saying, "Everyone seems to be too busy with their own lives to help me."

"I find negative thoughts running through my head day and night." What we say to ourselves about ourselves, our situation, and the future can create a tremendous amount of stress. In fact, many people find that their anticipation of what lies ahead is often more stressful than the actual tasks and that their negative thoughts intrude into the parts of the day when they could be enjoying their time. If this is the case, you need to work on recognizing the negative thoughts and replacing them with more realistic, posi-

tive ones. This will take practice, but it can be done. For example, instead of saying to yourself (perhaps over and over again), "I'm dreading tomorrow. I'll never be able to handle everything I'm expected to do," replace it with a more realistic statement, "I'm not looking forward to tomorrow, but I've handled days like this before and will be able to handle this one too." And try to keep your attention on the present, not the future.

But what if a careful analysis of your daily activities reveals that there is no way for you to cut back significantly on your responsibilities or to enlist the help of others? And what if you find that most of your negative thoughts about your situation are not exaggerated or unrealistic? There are still strategies that you can employ to reduce stress. One of the most important is to find someone you can trust and in whom you can confide your feelings about the difficulties in your life—a friend, a member of the clergy, a mental health professional, or members of a support group. Often during our most stressful times we are reluctant to let others know what we are going through, but that is exactly when we need to take the initiative to reach out and ask for help. You should not try to go through any sort of major stress—marital strife, financial difficulties, caring for an ill spouse—by yourself.

Something else to look for as you review your journal is whether or not you are still involved in activities that you find enjoyable and renewing. Often when we encounter stressful and demanding situations, the first thing we allow to drop from our schedule are activities that bring us pleasure and restore our spirits—listening to favorite music, reading interesting books, or taking leisurely walks. Granted, you may no longer have as much time as you did before to enjoy these activities, but with careful planning you should be able to find ways to get some of these back into your life. You should not underestimate the importance of these activities. We all need to provide this type of nourishment for ourselves.

Relaxation exercises are another tool that individuals can use to counteract some of the effects of stress. One of the commonly used approaches is "progressive muscle relaxation." In this method, you systematically tense different muscle groups and then gradually relax the muscles. You can start by tensing the muscles around your eyes for four or five seconds and then slowly releasing this tension until these muscles are completely relaxed. Next, tense the muscles around your mouth and jaw for a few seconds and then gradually release the tension until these muscles are relaxed. Follow this procedure for the other muscle groups, eventually moving all the way down to your feet and toes. While doing these exercises, be sure to keep your attention focused on the exercises themselves and to set aside any thoughts about your stressful situation.

Some people like to add to their progressive muscle relaxation exercises the technique of visualization. In this, you conjure up images of peaceful, relaxing situations—a calm, sunny day at the beach or a quiet, cool stroll in the park. For each image, try to imagine not only what you would see but also what you would hear and smell.

It is not always easy to achieve a relaxed state when your life is full of demanding responsibilities, but it can be done. The key is to practice your relaxation procedures regularly. Therefore, it is important to carve out of your schedule each day at least 15 minutes for practice.

Suggestions for Congregational Programs

- Offer classes in relaxation.
- Sponsor a stress management program offered by a mental health professional.
- Organize support groups or provide information about where individuals can find a support group.
- Offer a support group for caregivers, with respite care provided.

Information Resources

A tutorial prepared for MedlinePlus, a service of the U.S. National Library of Medicine and the National Institutes of Health, is available at www.nlm.nih.gov/medlineplus/tutorials/managingstress/htm/index.htm.

www.americanheart.org (American Heart Association)

www.familydoctor.org (American Academy of Family Physicians)

A BRIEF GUIDE TO INCREASING PHYSICAL ACTIVITY

One of the major risk factors for several serious medical conditions, including heart disease, stroke, and diabetes, is physical inactivity. Despite this well-documented link, the American Heart Association reports that nearly 40 percent of American adults over the age of 55 report no leisure-time physical activity. Clearly, there is a need for more programs to educate adults about the health benefits of increased physical activity and to provide ongoing encouragement and support for maintaining regular individualized programs of exercise.

Although regular exercise is safe for most adults, even those with chronic conditions, it is always advisable to check with your physician before embarking on a new exercise program. Once you have been cleared by your physician, you are ready to begin.

Getting started on a program of regular physical activity and then maintaining that program can be difficult. Many obstacles can interfere with our plans. To help people find strategies to overcome these barriers, the National Institute of Diabetes and Digestive and Kidney Diseases of the National Institutes of Health has prepared a booklet, *Tips to Help You Get Active*. This excellent booklet, available at www.win.niddk.nih.gov, is not copyrighted and can be duplicated. Here are some excerpts from this booklet:

BARRIER: Between work, family, and other demands, I am too busy to exercise.

> SOLUTIONS: Make physical activity a priority. Carve out some time each week to be active and put it on your calendar. Try waking up a half-hour earlier to walk, scheduling lunchtime workouts, or taking an evening fitness class.
>
> Build physical activity into your routine chores. Rake the yard, wash the car, or do energetic housework. That way you do what needs to be done and move around, too.
>
> Make family time physically active. Plan a weekend hike through a park, a family softball game, or an evening walk around the block.

BARRIER: By the end of a long day, I am just too tired to work out.

> SOLUTIONS: Break your workout into three 10-minute segments each

day. Taking three short walks during the day may seem easier and less tiring than one 30-minute workout and is just as good for you.

Find another time during the day to work out. If evening workouts are not for you, then try a bike ride before breakfast or a walk at lunchtime.

Sneak physical activity into your days. Take stairs instead of elevators, park further away in parking lots, and walk in place while watching television.

BARRIER: I think my weight is fine, so I am not motivated to exercise.

SOLUTIONS: Think about the other health benefits of physical activity. Regular physical activity may help lower cholesterol and blood pressure, and lower your odds of having heart disease, type 2 diabetes, or cancer. Research shows that people who are overweight, active, and fit live longer than people who are not overweight but are inactive and unfit. Also, physical activity may lift your mood and increase your energy level.

Do it just for fun. Play a team sport, work in a garden, or learn a new dance and make getting fit something fun.

Train for a charity event. You can work to help others while you work out.

BARRIER: Getting on a treadmill or stationary bike is boring.

SOLUTIONS: Meet a friend for workouts. If your buddy is on the next bike or treadmill, your workout will be less boring.

Watch television or listen to music or a book on tape while you walk or pedal indoors. Check out music or books on tape from your local library.

Get outside. A change in scenery can relieve your boredom. (If you are riding a bike outside, be sure to wear a helmet and learn safe rules of the road.)

BARRIER: I am afraid I will hurt myself.

SOLUTIONS: Start slowly. If you are starting a new physical activity program, go slow at the start. Even if you are doing an activity that you once did well, start up again slowly to lower your risk of injury or burnout.

Choose moderate-intensity physical activities. You are not likely to hurt yourself by walking 30 minutes per day. Doing vigorous physical activities may increase your risk for injury, but moderate-intensity physical activity is low risk.

Take a class. A knowledgeable group fitness instructor should be able to teach you how to move with proper form and lower risk for injury. The instructor can watch your actions during class and let you know if you are doing things right.

Choose water workouts. Whether you swim laps or try water aerobics, working out in the water is easy on your joints and helps reduce sore muscles and injury.

Work with a personal trainer. A certified personal trainer should be able to show you how to warm up, cool down, use fitness equipment like treadmills and weight-training machines, and use proper form to help lower your risk for injury. Personal training sessions may be cheap or costly, so find out about fees before making an appointment.

BARRIER: I have never been into sports.

SOLUTIONS: Find a physical activity that you enjoy. You do not have to be an athlete to benefit from physical activity. Try yoga, hiking, or planting a garden.

Choose an activity that you can stick with, like walking. Just put one foot in front of the other. Use the time you spend walking to relax, talk with a friend or family member, or just enjoy the scenery.

BARRIER: I do not want to spend a lot of money to join a gym or buy workout gear.

SOLUTIONS: Choose free activities. Garden, take your children to the park to play, lift plastic milk jugs filled with water or sand, or take a walk.

Find out if your job offers any discounts on memberships. Some companies get lower membership rates at fitness or community centers. Other companies will even pay for part of an employee's membership fee.

Check out your local recreation or community center. These centers may cost less than other gyms, fitness centers, or health clubs.

Choose physical activities that do not require any special gear. Walking requires only a pair of sturdy shoes. To dance, just turn on some music.

BARRIER: I do not have anyone to watch my kids while I work out.

SOLUTIONS: Do something physically active with your kids. Kids need physical activity too. No matter what age your kids are, you can find an activity you can do together. Dance to music, take a walk, run around the park, or play basketball or soccer together.

Take turns with another parent to watch the kids. One of you minds the kids while the other one works out.

Hire a baby-sitter.

Look for a fitness or community center that offers childcare. Centers that have childcare are becoming more popular. Cost and quality vary, so get all the information up front.

BARRIER: My family and friends are not physically active.

SOLUTIONS: Do not let that stop you. Do it for yourself. Enjoy the rewards—such as better sleep, a happier mood, more energy, and a stronger body—you get from working out.

Join a class or sports league where people count on you to show up. If your basketball team or dance partner counts on you, you will not want to miss a workout, even if your family and friends are not involved.

BARRIER: I would be embarrassed if my neighbors or friends saw me exercising.

SOLUTIONS: Ask yourself if it really matters. You are doing something positive for your health, and that is something to be proud of. You may even inspire others to get physically active too.

Invite a friend or neighbor to join you. You may feel less self-conscious if you are not alone.

Go to a park, nature trail, or fitness or community center to be physically active.

BARRIER: My neighborhood does not have sidewalks.

SOLUTIONS: Find a safe place to walk. Instead of walking in the street, walk in a friend or family member's neighborhood that has sidewalks. Walk during your lunch break at work. Find out if you can walk at a local school track.

Work out in the yard. Do yard work or wash the car. These count as physical activity.

BARRIER: The winter is too cold/summer is too hot to be active outdoors.

SOLUTIONS: Walk around the mall.

Join a fitness or community center. Find one that lets you pay only for the months or classes you want, instead of the whole year.

Exercise at home. Work out to fitness videos or DVDs. Check out a different one from the library each week for variety.

BARRIER: I do not feel safe exercising by myself.

SOLUTIONS: Join or start a walking group. You can enjoy added safety and company as you walk.

Take an exercise class at a nearby fitness or community center.

Work out at home. You don't need a lot of space. Turn on the radio and dance or follow along with a fitness show on TV.

BARRIER: I have a health problem (diabetes, heart disease, asthma, arthritis) that I do not want to make worse.

SOLUTIONS: Talk with your health care professional. Most health problems are helped by physical activity. Find out what physical activities you can safely do and follow advice about length and intensity of workouts.

Start slowly. Take it easy at first and see how you feel before trying more challenging workouts. Stop if you feel out of breath, dizzy, faint, or nauseated, or if you have pain.

BARRIER: I have an injury and do not know what physical activities, if any, I can do.

SOLUTIONS: Talk with your health care professional. Ask your physician or physical therapist about what physical activities you can safely perform. Follow advice about length and intensity of workouts.

Start slowly. Take it easy at first and see how you feel before trying more challenging workouts. Stop if you feel pain.

Work with a personal trainer. A knowledgeable personal trainer should be able to help you design a fitness plan around your injury.

SUGGESTIONS FOR CONGREGATIONAL PROGRAMS

- Sponsor a workshop on exercise led by a physical therapist.
- Organize groups into friendly competition (e.g., which group can accumulate the most distance walked during a certain period?).
- Create a list for members who are looking for partners to join them

in a program of regular physical activity (e.g., walking or biking together).

• Organize a walking group.

Information Resources

www.win.niddk.nih.gov (Weight-control Information Network, an information service of the National Institute of Diabetes and Digestive and Kidney Diseases)

www.cdc.gov (Centers for Disease Control and Prevention)

www.americanheart.org (American Heart Association)

A BRIEF GUIDE TO LOSING WEIGHT

The most common approach to weight loss has been dieting, a method in which people focus on restricting their caloric intake. Although the basic equation underlying this approach is correct—weight loss results when the calories you use exceed the calories you take in—the weight loss produced by using this approach alone is generally not maintained for long. A more effective strategy for weight loss is a multidimensional approach that can be incorporated into your overall lifestyle and sustained for the rest of your life.

The first step is to assess your readiness to initiate a weight reduction program. What is your motivation for trying to lose weight? Are you clear about the health risks of maintaining your current weight and the benefits of losing weight? Have you checked with your physician in order to set a reasonable goal and to get advice about any specific dietary concerns? Have you thought about how to enlist the support of your family and friends?

The next step is to carefully monitor and record your eating habits: What do you eat? How much of each food do you eat? When do you eat? Where do you eat? Do you eat more when people are around, or when you are by yourself? Are your eating habits when dining out different from those at home? Which setting is more challenging? Be as specific as possible. It is also helpful to record any situations or emotions that trigger your desire to eat. For example, do you eat when you are lonely or anxious? You should plan on continuing to monitor your eating habits as you implement your weight reduction program. This will enable you to identify new obstacles and then make appropriate adjustments.

After you have analyzed the various aspects of your eating habits, you need to take the time to begin developing a plan that addresses the problem areas you have identified. The goal is to come up with practical strategies that will make it easier for you to cut back on your caloric intake. Some possible aspects of a plan may be readily apparent. For example, if you discovered that you find it hard not to snack when there are cookies or other high-calorie items in your kitchen cabinet, you should purchase fewer of these high-calorie items and more healthful, low-calorie items. (Helpful hint: Most people find it easier to pass up tasty, high-calorie items in the grocery store if they do their shopping immediately after they have had a satisfying meal. Also, make up your grocery list in advance and stick to it.) If you get hungry sometimes while working and the only food available at your worksite are high-calorie snacks, you can prepare for this by purchasing or preparing some low-calorie snacks to take with you. Or if you find that you tend to snack when you are lonely, substitute an alternative activity—perhaps calling a friend or going for a walk.

If you find that you tend to overeat when you are dining out, you can cut back on the frequency of dining out, or you can opt instead to reduce the amount of food you eat in restaurants. Although leaving food on your plate may run counter to what you learned as a child, it is an important part of losing weight, especially because the portions served by many restaurants are quite large. And there is always the option of asking for a "doggy bag" and saving part of your dinner for another meal.

Another useful strategy to employ, no matter where you are eating, is to pay more attention to the actual eating process. The goal here is to eat less but enjoy it more. One way to do this is to eat more slowly and focus on savoring each bite or mouthful, enjoying the taste and texture of your food. Record how long it typically takes you to eat your meal and then work on gradually lengthening this period. If you find it difficult to eat more slowly, try putting down your eating utensils after every few mouthfuls. This generally slows eating and reduces the total amount of food consumed.

Physical activity needs to be a part of your weight-reduction plan. This can take many forms—walking, biking, jogging, swimming, aerobic exercise classes, and so on. The best strategy is to choose an activity you enjoy and then add it to your daily routine. Most experts recommend 30 minutes of moderate-intensity physical activity five or more days a week. If you find it hard to carve a 30-minute block out of your schedule, then break it down into shorter blocks of time. Three 10-minute periods devoted to physical activity burn as many calories as one 30-minute period. Another good strategy, and one that yields double benefits, is to go for a walk during a break at work or a time at home when you normally would have a snack.

Changing eating habits is always a challenge, and especially so if you do not have the support of family and friends. Therefore, it is important to enlist the assistance of as many as you can. Explain to family, friends, and co-workers what you are trying to accomplish and why it is important. Give them specific suggestions for how they can help you. For example, ask family members to cooperate with you when planning meals and snacks at home and shopping for groceries. If you find it easier to exercise regularly when you have a partner, ask a friend to join you. When your friends or co-workers are deciding which restaurant to go to, request that they choose one that has options that are on your diet.

As you design your weight-reduction program, set reasonable goals. Remember, the objective is not to have a quick, dramatic loss of weight but to reach a healthy weight that you can sustain for the rest of your life. This means that you should strive for modest losses every week or so. Set reasonable goals for implementing the changes in your routine. You do not have to tackle every problem area at once. Pick one aspect of your plan (e.g., eating more slowly) and focus on implementing it successfully before moving on to the next one.

As part of your program, establish a system of rewards for achieving your goals. Make a list of several items you would like to purchase for yourself and link each to one of your goals, or think of events and activities you would enjoy and make your participation in these events and activities contingent on achieving certain goals. You can even use dining at your favorite restaurant as a reward.

Finally, prepare for occasional setbacks. Even with the best of intentions and a well-designed weight-reduction program, you may not find it possible to always adhere to your program. When these lapses occur, do not make the mistake of giving up. View lapses as learning experiences, not as failures. Carefully review what happened and think of ways you can handle similar situations should they occur.

Suggestions for Congregational Programs

- Sponsor a workshop on healthy eating and weight reduction led by a dietitian.
- Organize a support group for individuals interested in losing weight.
- Provide information about weight-reduction programs in the community.

Information Resources

www.win.niddk.nih.gov (Weight-control Information Network, an information service of the National Institute of Diabetes and Digestive and Kidney Diseases)

www.cdc.gov (Centers for Disease Control and Prevention)

www.diabetes.org (American Diabetes Association)

A BRIEF GUIDE TO SMOKING CESSATION

Smoking is the number one cause of preventable death in America. Estimates are that about half of the people who do not quit smoking will die of smoking-related problems. Individuals who smoke have an increased risk of cancer, lung disease, heart attack, stroke, vascular disease, and even blindness. In spite of the well-documented link between smoking and these serious medical conditions, many people find it extremely difficult to quit smoking. The primary reason underlying this difficulty is the addictive nature of nicotine.

Although stopping smoking can be difficult, the health benefits for those who succeed are significant and well worth the effort. For example, after one year your risk of a heart attack drops by 50 percent, and after five years your risk of a stroke is the same as that of a nonsmoker.

Knowing how difficult it is to stop smoking, individuals who decide to quit first need to develop a plan that takes into account the obstacles they are likely to encounter and the resources available to help them overcome these obstacles. This process starts by assessing your readiness. What is your motivation for stopping? What is likely to happen if you do not stop? What are the benefits if you can? When listing benefits, start with the positive impact this will have on your health (e.g., living longer, reducing your risk of having a heart attack, stroke, cancer, and lung disease), but be sure to include the benefits it will have on others (e.g., reducing their risk of diseases associated with second-hand smoke) and the financial benefits for you and your family as you spend less on tobacco products. Keep this list in a place where you can review it regularly.

Think through your daily routine and identify the various challenges you will face and the resources that are available. In what situations will the temptation to smoke be the greatest? What events are likely to trigger the urge to smoke? Has smoking been one of the ways you typically respond to stress or feelings of depression? If you have tried to stop smoking before, review how you approached the challenge then and what interfered with your attempt(s). What can you do differently this time? Who are the people most likely to discourage or interfere with your effort to quit smoking? Who are the individuals you will definitely be able to count on to support your effort?

As you begin to develop your smoking cessation plan, consult with your physician and inquire about the medications that have been approved to help people stop smoking. Studies have shown that taking these medications can double your chance of success. Make sure you understand how to use the medication and what the side effects might be. You also can ask if your physician knows of any hospital-sponsored smoking cessation programs or behavioral health professionals (e.g., psychologists or other mental health professionals) who specialize in working with individuals who are trying to stop smoking. If there are no programs or professionals in your community, telephone counseling is available at 1-800-QUIT-NOW.

The next step is to share your decision to quit and your motivation for quitting with family and friends. Request their support, offering them specific suggestions when you can. For example, ask those who smoke not to do so around you and those who do not smoke, especially the ones who did at one time but were able to quit, to provide encouragement for your efforts.

Because people often use smoking as a method of coping with stress, you may want to practice some stress management techniques before you stop smoking. Also build time and opportunities for more physical activity into your smoking cessation plan. This can help reduce stress and can also burn some of the extra calories if you find yourself eating more when you stop smoking.

Making changes in your home and work environment can help. Discard or move out of sight ashtrays and other items associated with smoking. Plan on changing your daily routine as well, and be sure to include pleasurable activities, especially ones that can help distract you when you have the urge to smoke.

Once you have identified the various challenges you will face, devised strategies for meeting these challenges, and pulled together the social resources (e.g., family, friends, and co-workers) and medical resources (e.g., medication) you will need, you are ready to stop smoking. The first few weeks are likely to be difficult, so during this time be sure to make good use of all the strategies and resources you have included in your plan (e.g., regularly review your list of reasons for stopping, spend time with your nonsmoking friends, stay active). You also need to be prepared for setbacks—difficult or stressful situations where you are unable to resist the urge to smoke. If these occur, do not become discouraged and give up on your plan to quit smoking. Relapses are fairly common, even among highly motivated individuals and do not mean that you will not be successful eventually. Use each setback as a learning experience and an opportunity to improve your plan. What situational or emotional cues seemed to trigger the smoking? How could you avoid these cues or handle them more effectively? Then start again. Remember, the benefits of giving up smoking are so great that it is worth repeated efforts.

Suggestions for Congregational Programs

- Disseminate information about local smoking-cessation programs.
- Sponsor a seminar on medications approved to help people stop smoking.

Information Resources

www.smokefree.gov (Tobacco Control Research Branch of the National Cancer Institute)
www.cdc.gov (Centers for Disease Control and Prevention)
www.acs.org (American Cancer Society)
www.lungusa.org (American Lung Association)

EXAMPLES OF CONGREGATIONAL PROGRAMS

The health ministry program at College Park Baptist Church in Orlando, Florida, illustrates the tremendous impact a dedicated volunteer can have on the health of a congregation, especially when she has the strong support of her minister. After completing her training in the lay health education program sponsored by Florida Hospital, Barbara Pearson worked closely with her pastor, Dr. Charles Horton, and staff from Florida Hospital to create a comprehensive health education program. To "kick off" the program, Dr. Horton preached a sermon, "The Theology of Health," in which he focused on the importance of being good stewards of one of God's greatest gifts—our bodies. He voiced his own commitment to taking better care of his body—exercising regularly and eating wisely—and encouraged members to make a similar commitment. This was followed by a series of health education seminars held on Wednesday evenings.

Several of the programs focused on risk factors for cardiovascular diseases and diabetes. For example, an exercise physiologist from the hospital gave a presentation on strategies and suggestions for increasing physical activity and then answered questions from the audience. Another part of this series, this one spread over three weekly meetings, focused on the important role of diet. These seminars were led by a dietitian from the hospital. For one seminar, she discussed the U.S. Department of Agriculture's recently revised food pyramid, a food guidance system that helps people design their own nutritional program. For a second seminar, she conducted a cooking demonstration, and in the third seminar she provided examples of how to cook healthy meals for the entire family. For this seminar, bag lunches that were both healthy and fun for kids were given out.

An example of religious congregations partnering with health care professionals, medical institutions, and other community organizations to promote health and prevent chronic diseases by teaching people to modify risk factors is found in the work of La Vaida Owens-White, M.S.N., R.N. Ms. Owens-White is employed by Christiana Care Health System in Delaware and serves as Faith Community Nurse for the Helen F. Graham Cancer Center's Community Outreach and Education program. She is also a member of the City of Wilmington's Health Planning Committee.

Ms. Owens-White has worked with several congregations to establish health ministries focused on chronic disease prevention. One of the programs she developed for her own congregation illustrates how this can be done. Well aware of the important role physical activity can play in promoting health and preventing disease, she and the health ministry team at Christ our King Catholic Church initiated a virtual "Walk to Jerusalem." Ms. Owens-White had learned of a similar program developed by St. John Health Parish Nursing in Detroit, Michigan, while attending one of the Health Ministries Association's annual conferences. She began by purchasing pedometers to record participants' daily steps. Although their virtual journey took longer than initially expected, they eventually did meet their goal. They have continued this program each year, and participation has increased. She has found that at the conclusion of their virtual journey each year, participants continue in an exercise program of some kind (e.g., walking, swimming, housework activities, etc.), and recently they decided to expand their health promotion program to include units on nutrition and weight management.

14

MANAGING MEDICATIONS

Even adults who have no outward signs of ill health can take many prescribed and over-the-counter medications to treat common conditions such as high blood pressure, high cholesterol, acid reflux, and arthritis. As individuals age and develop chronic diseases, the list of medications frequently grows long. In a 2007 "Personal Health" column in the *New York Times,* Jane E. Brody referred to the "poisonous cocktail" of multiple drugs, and geriatricians have long referred to the multiplicity of drugs prescribed to older patients—often by multiple specialists—as *polypharmacy.* In the early 1990s, federal regulators required that nursing home residents taking more than nine medications—then considered a large number—be identified and evaluated for possible overmedication. Ironically, in more recent years so many residents of long-term care facilities are taking this number of medications or more that this recommendation may now apply to a majority of nursing home residents. Regardless of the number of medications any one person takes, adverse side effects are always possible, and the risks increase dramatically as the number of medications rises.

Acute illnesses related to adverse drug reactions may account for up to a quarter of the hospitalizations in the United States each year, and some experts estimate that adverse drug reactions are among the top ten causes of death. A recent article in the *Annals of Internal Medicine* noted that visits to the emergency department occurred regularly for adverse drug reactions related to three commonly prescribed medications: warfarin (Coumadin), insulin, and digoxin (Budnitz, Shehab, Kegler, and Richards 2007).

Although adverse reactions to medications occur frequently, noncompliance with prescribed regimens, especially medications, is probably even more common. Studies have shown that as many as 50 percent of patients fail to take their medications as prescribed. The problem is even greater for older adults, in large part because they are likely to have multiple chronic diseases and thus are prescribed many medications.

Numerous factors contribute to the high incidence of noncompliance, and many can be traced to communication problems between patients and physicians. Often patients do not understand why their doctor has prescribed a certain medication. They may not understand its use and benefits and may not be aware of the risks of not taking the medication as prescribed. Unpleasant side effects sometimes lead to noncompliance. Frequently patients who experience unpleasant side effects stop taking the medication without informing their physicians. Noncompliance also increases as the number of medications prescribed increases. Because elderly persons take an average of five to seven medications, it is not surprising that many have difficulty organizing and taking all of their medications as prescribed.

Finally, noncompliance can be related to economic status. Some medications are quite expensive, and individuals with limited financial resources may be forced to choose between buying a prescribed medicine and purchasing another needed product or service.

THE RISKS OF IGNORING INFORMATION ON MEDICATION MANAGEMENT

The most serious danger of failing to take a medication as instructed is that the disorder or condition for which it is prescribed will not be controlled and thus an individual will be at risk of developing more serious medical problems. For example, people with hypertension who fail to take their antihypertensive medication on a regular basis are increasing their chances of having a stroke or heart attack. Another danger is that if people take some medications improperly, they may develop new medical problems, such as mental confusion or injuries sustained from a fall because of an imbalance related to adverse effects on brain function. Finally, even if medications are taken properly, adverse drug reactions can occur. Therefore, it is important for patients to understand the most frequent symptoms to watch for when beginning a new medication and to always investigate with their physician or pharmacist whether new symptoms might be related to the medication they are taking.

Below is a brief guide we have prepared to help people manage their prescription and nonprescription medications. This guide can be copied and distributed to interested persons. It is also available in PDF format on the Web site of the O'Neill Foundation for Community Health (www.oneill communityhealth.org) and can be downloaded and copied.

MANAGING MEDICATIONS

Medications can generally be managed effectively if you follow these recommendations:

- Understand why the physician has prescribed a medication. If you do not understand, you should ask. You should know what the medication is for, how to take it, and what to expect, including understanding common side effects or conditions that should prompt you to contact your physician.
- Write down the information and instructions provided by your physician. You should take notes about the prescribed medication while you are in the doctor's office. (The form in appendix F can be used to assist with this.)
- Keep an up-to-date list of all current prescription and nonprescription medications as well as any dietary or herbal supplements being taken, and bring this list to all physician appointments and to the pharmacy when having any new prescription filled. This list should be available to family members or other caregivers. In the event of an emergency, this list can be referred to by health care providers.
- Ask about foods and drinks that should be avoided while taking the medication(s).
- Ask your primary care physician to review all of your medications. Take your medications, or at least a list of all your medications, to office visits. Over-the-counter (nonprescription) drugs, dietary supplements, and herbal remedies should be included.
- Report any unexpected or unpleasant side effects to your doctor.
- Use one pharmacist or pharmacy for all of your medications and accept medication counseling when it is offered by a pharmacist. If you still have any questions about the medication, ask your phar-

macist or physician. In fact, pharmacists are required by law to offer medication counseling whenever a prescription is dispensed.

- Ask your pharmacist to contact your doctor if you feel you cannot afford the medication that has been prescribed. The pharmacist and physician may be able to find a less expensive alternative.
- Take a relative or friend with you if you have difficulty talking with your physician or pharmacist.
- Use medication organizers or pill boxes if you have trouble remembering your medicine. These inexpensive boxes can be purchased at pharmacies, or you can construct your own.
- Keep a record of your medications. This should include information about the drug, what it is for, its color and shape, directions and cautions, and the times at which it should be taken. (Appendix F provides a sample medication record.)

SUGGESTIONS FOR CONGREGATIONAL PROGRAMS

Sponsor a program or series of programs on medication management with a local pharmacist as the featured speaker. Among the topics that could be covered in a series on medications are communicating with your pharmacist and physician about medications; commonly prescribed drugs and common mistakes people make when taking these medications; and non-prescription medications.

Schedule a meeting about medications. Encourage members of your congregation to put all their medications, including nonprescription medications, dietary supplements, and herbal remedies, in a bag and bring them to the meeting. Have a pharmacist available to meet privately with members to review and discuss the various medications.

Provide members of your congregation with medication record forms. These are easy and simple to design or copy. (Appendix F provides a sample form.)

Offer members of your congregation medication organizers. The organizers can be purchased at pharmacies or on-line, or constructed by volunteers. Some hospitals and pharmaceutical companies may be willing to donate a small number of the organizers.

Use congregational bulletins and mailings to remind members of your congregation of the need to take their medications as directed. Information on some of the more commonly prescribed medications, which can be obtained from the local hospital or pharmacies, can be included.

EXAMPLES OF CONGREGATIONAL PROGRAMS

An informative program on medication management was coordinated by volunteers from four churches in the greater Daytona Beach community. All Saints Lutheran, Grace Episcopal, Westminster by-the-Sea Presbyterian, and Christian and Missionary Alliance sponsored a Saturday morning program on several topics, including medications. In spite of rain and severe weather warnings, more than forty people attended. The first part of the program, held in the sanctuary of All Saints Lutheran Church, consisted of presentations by a panel of health care professionals. Panelists included a pharmacist, a physician, a dietitian, and a physical therapist. Members of the audience were encouraged to ask the panelists questions or to write their questions on a card and have the moderator direct the questions to the appropriate panelist. Several questions on medications were asked, and it proved quite helpful to have not only a pharmacist but also a physician and a dietitian available to respond to different issues related to medications.

For the second part of the program, each professional was given a classroom in the education wing of the church, and members of the audience were invited to participate in small group or individual discussions with the health professionals. Most of the audience stayed for this part and took advantage of the opportunity to talk with health care professionals in a setting that was more relaxed and less hurried than the typical office or pharmacy visit.

Another excellent educational program on medication management was held as part of a five-week health education series sponsored by College Park Baptist Church in Orlando, Florida. Each Wednesday night during the month of January, members were invited to attend these sessions, which began immediately after the regularly scheduled church supper. Almost a hundred members attended the session on medications. This program was held in the chapel and featured Timothy Regan, a pharmacist from Florida Hospital, as the guest speaker. He received an enthusiastic introduction by Barbara Pearson, the lay health educator. She first became acquainted with him when he led her lay health educator training workshop on medication management, and she knew that the audience would find him as interesting and informative as she had.

Mr. Regan emphasized several points during his presentation, but the overarching message was that people need to take responsibility for understanding their medications. In discussing their medications with their doctor and pharmacist people need to take the initiative, and they should not be shy about asking questions. He encouraged the members of the congregation to take their medications, or at least a complete list of their medications (including over-the-counter medications), to their visits with their doctor or to the pharmacy when getting a new prescription filled. In addition, he suggested that they keep a chart describing their medications, what they are for, and when they should be taken. (Sample charts were provided for those who were interested.) He also repeatedly emphasized that they should not hesitate to call their pharmacist whenever they had a question about their medications.

During the question-and-answer session that followed, Mr. Regan was asked several questions about specific medications, including generic drugs. The audience seemed enthusiastic about his presentation and thanked both him and the lay health educator for offering the program.

INFORMATION RESOURCES

The National Council on Patient Information and Education, a coalition of consumer organizations, health care organizations, government agencies, and business organizations, has a number of educational materials that can be ordered from the organization's Web site (www.talkaboutrx.org). Also available as a free download is the form, "Make Notes and Take Notes," a guide to help people avoid medication errors.

The Food and Drug Administration has consumer education materials on its Web site (www.fda.gov/cder/consumerinfo/DPAdefault .htm).

Local pharmacies can supply information sheets on various medications.

15

ACCIDENTS AND FALLS

Accidents and falls frequently are overlooked as major health problems associated with aging. However, both the incidence and the severity of falls increase with age, and accidents are among the ten leading causes of death among older adults. Almost one-third of adults aged 65 or older who live at home experience falls each year. Approximately one in forty of these falls results in hospitalization.

Many factors increase the risk of falls among older adults. Some of these, including changes in postural control and gait, are associated with the aging process. Other factors are associated with medical disorders (e.g., diabetes or stroke) that occur more frequently in old age. Such disorders can cause muscle weakness, sensory deficits, or balance problems that can lead to instability. In addition, adverse reactions to many commonly prescribed medications can result in inattention, drowsiness, dizziness, or weakness and can directly cause a fall. Finally, many falls are the result of environmental factors that could be prevented if proper home inspections and modifications are made.

THE RISKS OF IGNORING INFORMATION ON ACCIDENTS AND FALLS

Complications of falls include fractures and neurological injuries that frequently result in serious functional limitations. People who have fallen and suffered injuries may experience permanent problems with mobility. In addition, the fear of falling that often follows a major injury may result in curtailment of activities, leading to muscle weakening and, paradoxically, possibly further increasing the risk of future falls. People who fall likely will experience a loss of independence and are at greater risk of being institutionalized.

WHAT CAN BE DONE TO REDUCE THE RISK OF ACCIDENTS AND FALLS?

Fortunately, patients, their families, and caregivers can make a number of changes in the living environments of older adults to reduce the risk of accidents and falls, such as:

Removing throw rugs
Tacking down large rugs and carpeting completely
Removing furniture that is low to the ground or likely to move
Keeping objects off the floor
Using nonslip polish on floors
Installing handrails along both sides of stairs
Providing good lighting on steps, landings, and any other particularly
    dark areas
Placing light switches in easily accessible locations near doors and
    room entrances
Using nightlights in bedrooms, bathrooms, and hallways
Using nonskid rubber mats in showers or baths
Installing handrails for baths and toilets
Keeping water off the floors
Using adaptive equipment for baths or showers (e.g., seats or
    benches)
Installing raised toilet seats or using a bedside commode
Keeping food and other necessary items on low, easy-to-reach
    shelves

People also can reduce the risk of accidents and falls by using assistive devices such as canes or walkers. Medical professionals and therapists need to encourage people who would benefit from such devices to use the most appropriate and effective ones, and to emphasize how they can help to prevent falls and serious, even life-threatening, injuries.

SUGGESTIONS FOR CONGREGATIONAL PROGRAMS

Sponsor a program on home safety, mobility, and assistive devices. A physical therapist could be one of your featured speakers, along with representatives from several companies that provide in-home medical supplies and equipment.

Recruit and train a group of volunteers who would be willing to conduct home safety checks for members of the congregation. Social workers from the local hospital or a home health agency can assist in their training.

Recruit and train a group of volunteers who are willing to use their knowledge and skills to make minor modifications based on home safety checks (e.g., install grab bars and handrails).

Recruit and train a group of volunteers who are willing to deliver meals or provide basic home services (e.g., cleaning, laundry, etc.) *to people with physical limitations.* This service could help some individuals avoid or delay placement in a nursing home or other long-term care facility.

Organize a group of volunteers who are willing to provide basic house and yard maintenance for people who are physically incapacitated. This could be done on a short- or long-term basis, depending on the congregation's needs and resources. Seasonal activities such as lawn mowing, leaf raking, snow shoveling, or spring gardening help might be organized.

Use congregational bulletins and mailings to provide members with helpful suggestions and reminders about home safety. Home health agencies, companies that provide in-home medical supplies and equipment, or advocacy organizations (e.g., National Stroke Association, American Stroke Association) may have materials that you can distribute.

EXAMPLES OF CONGREGATIONAL PROGRAMS

A congregational program designed to reduce accidents and injuries was coordinated by two lay health educators at First Baptist Church in DeLand, Florida. They began by inserting in the church's bulletin and also in its newsletter, which is mailed to all members of the church, a list of suggestions on how to reduce the risk of accidents in the home. Accompanying this list was an announcement of a special program on the same topic that would be given during the next regularly scheduled meeting of the church's seniors group. They also invited members of nearby churches and a retirement center to attend the program. A gerontologist from the local college was the featured speaker, and a physical therapist from the local hospital was available to answer questions. In addition, the lay health educators and several other members of the church offered to conduct home safety checks and modifications for older adults who needed assistance.

Another program designed to reduce accidents and injuries was sponsored by the O'Neill Foundation for Community Health (see chapter 17) and Florida Hospital DeLand. Invitations to attend this free program, titled "Fall Prevention and Safety in the Home," were mailed to all religious congregations in DeLand and the surrounding community, and an announcement was placed in the religion section of the local newspaper. The program, held at a downtown church, attracted an audience of 60 and featured two physical therapists (one from the hospital's rehabilitation department and the other from the hospital's home health agency), a pharmacist, and a representative of a medical equipment company.

The program began with the physical therapist from the home health agency reviewing various safety hazards in the home and offering suggestions for removing or avoiding these hazards. She was followed by the physical therapist from the rehabilitation department, who demonstrated exercises individuals could do in their homes to gain strength and improve their balance. The representative of the medical equipment company then demonstrated a number of assistive devices and types of mobility equipment, including canes, walkers, rollators, transfer benches, scooters, and power chairs. The final presentation was by a pharmacist who reviewed the various types of medications that could increase the risk of falling. The presenters then fielded questions from the audience and also remained after the conclusion of the program to meet with several individuals who had additional questions.

INFORMATION RESOURCES

Information and materials on preventing falls and accidents can be found on the Web site of the Centers for Disease Control and Prevention's National Center for Injury Prevention and Control (www .cdc.gov/ncipc/duip/spotlite/falls.htm).

The National Institute on Aging (NIA) also has materials on preventing falls that can be ordered or downloaded from NIA's Web site (www.niapublications.org/agepages/falls.asp).

Resources for programs on home safety can often be found in local institutions and agencies. Hospitals, home health agencies, and medical equipment companies can provide materials for your programs and help you find professionals who can serve as guest speakers.

III

RESOURCES

16

COMMUNITY RESOURCES

Many chronic conditions and serious injuries can create significant challenges for people who want to maintain their independence. If they do not have family or friends who can step in to assist them physically or handle some of the everyday tasks and responsibilities required to live independently in the community, they may find it necessary to move to another setting. Even if a person has a spouse or someone to live with, eventually he or she may face the prospect of moving to a less independent setting as a condition progresses. For individuals who are faced with these situations but prefer to stay in their own homes as long as possible, the key may be finding professionals and agencies in the community that can provide help. Because arranging such services can be a daunting challenge for individuals who are already ill or injured, members of a faith community can help in several ways.

The easiest step for a faith community is to create and regularly update a list of community resources, including a brief description of the services provided and contact information for local agencies. In addition, the congregation can sponsor seminars or health fairs at which agencies share information about their services. These programs give members of the congregation and community an opportunity to learn about community resources *before* they or family members need the services. Finally, members in some congregations, particularly those who have a background in health care or social services, may provide direct assistance to ill or injured individuals by taking on some of their everyday responsibilities or chores (e.g., transportation, shopping, etc.), perhaps organizing groups or teams that can share these responsibilities.

Developing a list of community resources can be done by telephone and on the Internet. A good way to begin is to contact the case management or social work department of your local hospital. The professionals in these departments are generally aware of the various services in the community. They should be able to provide you with a list of many of the services and programs, along with information about which services are likely to be covered by Medicare or other insurance policies and the typical eligibility requirements for coverage.

Your Area Agency on Aging can be a source of information about community services. Established by the Older Americans Act of 1965, these Area Agencies on Aging (there are 650 across the country) provide home- and community-based services to older adults, thus allowing them to remain in their home. They also provide support services for caregivers. To locate the Area Agency on Aging for your community, you can call 1-800-677-1116 or go to the Eldercare locator (www.eldercare.gov/Eldercare .NET/Public/Home.aspx).

Another good source of information about community agencies and programs is your local chapter of the United Way. Each chapter has a list of affiliates or partner agencies, many of which offer services for individuals with functional impairment. The location of your local United Way chapter can be found by going to www.unitedway.org. Many United Way chapters are involved in establishing and supporting the 2-1-1 telephone program. In communities with this program, people can call 2-1-1 to obtain information about health and human services. Services vary from community to community but often include food banks, rent assistance, utility assistance, support groups, transportation assistance, Meals on Wheels, respite care, adult day care, and homemaker services.

An additional source of information about services in many communities is the local chapter of AARP. This organization also offers materials on a number of topics individuals and families with disease- or injury-related limitations are likely to encounter. Among the topics offered are caregiving, home modification to improve safety, housing choices, legal issues, and driver safety. You can obtain these materials and information about your state and local chapters by visiting the AARP's Web site: www.aarp.org.

The consumer beneficiary Web site offered by Medicare (www.medi care.gov) has information about health-related services in your community. This site allows you to list and compare the hospitals, skilled nursing facilities (nursing homes), home health agencies, health plans and Medigap policies, and suppliers of medical equipment by state, county, or even Zip code.

TRANSPORTATION

One of the problems facing many individuals who have functional limitations and are living alone is transportation. They may be unable to drive themselves to medical appointments or to do basic shopping, and their health-related limitations may prevent them from using regular public transportation. In many communities the public transportation agency is able to provide door-to-door transportation for such individuals. Members of a congregational health ministry team can contact your local transportation agency to see if this service is offered in your community and, if so, how this transportation can be arranged. This information may also be available through your local Area Agency on Aging. Additionally, some home care or personal care agencies offer transportation services. Experienced case managers also suggest contacting a dialysis center and inquiring about the transportation services their clients use.

ASSISTIVE DEVICES

People with functional limitations are often able to continue living in their homes and maintain much of their independence if they have appropriate assistive devices. These can include grab bars in the bathroom, bath and shower chairs, hand-held shower heads, raised toilet seats, transfer benches, bed grips, and lift chairs or lift cushions. Mobility aids, ranging from canes and walkers to motorized wheelchairs, can also help people maintain their functional independence. The congregational health ministry team can help individuals experiencing functional limitations by creating a list of local businesses that sell or rent this equipment. If local businesses do not carry all the items people need, there is the option of finding online businesses that have a comprehensive inventory of assistive devices. A related service that a congregation can offer is sponsoring a program at which an occupational therapist or other health professional familiar with assistive devices can demonstrate their proper usage.

HOME MODIFICATIONS

It may be necessary in some cases for individuals to modify certain features of their home if they are to continue living there. A ramp may need to be installed if they are using a wheelchair or have difficulty climbing steps, and doorways may need to be widened to accommodate a walker or wheelchair. The installation of better lighting and handrails, along with the removal of throw rugs, can reduce the risk of falls. Congregational health ministry team members can help by identifying contractors who have experience making these types of modifications. A good place to find these contractors is a local medical supply business that carries assistive devices and other durable medical equipment.

PERSONAL EMERGENCY RESPONSE SYSTEMS

A personal emergency response system, also called a medical response emergency system or medical alert system, can provide a sense of security for individuals living alone. These systems allow persons who are experiencing an emergency to summon help by simply pressing a button on a small radio transmitter carried in their pocket or worn around their neck or on their wrist. This sends a signal to a console connected to the user's telephone that automatically dials 911 or an emergency response center. With the systems that are linked to an emergency response center, the operator determines the nature of the emergency and notifies the appropriate party from a list provided by the client (e.g., neighbor, family member, ambulance). Some emergency response centers are operated by hospitals or social service agencies; others are operated by the system manufacturer. Members of a congregational health ministry team can research the options available in their community and the cost of renting or purchasing a personal emergency response system. In many communities, the Area Agency on Aging can arrange for the installation of a system or provide information about local providers. Also, businesses that sell or rent home medical equipment generally have information about these systems.

Individuals who have mobile telephones should consider creating one or more entries using the acronym ICE—In Case of Emergency—to assist paramedics or police who might need to alert a family member or friend in case of an emergency. The acronym can be placed in front of the name of the person or persons they would want called if they are in an emergency and unable to communicate. For example, they might have ICE–wife and ICE–son or ICE–1 and ICE–2. This would allow the paramedic or police to quickly notify the appropriate family member or friend.

MEAL PROGRAMS

Meals on Wheels is a nation-wide program that provides meals for homebound individuals unable to prepare their own meals. Information about local programs can be obtained from the Web site of Meals on Wheels Association of America (www.mowaa.org) or from your Area Agency on Aging. Many communities also offer congregate dining programs for older adults who have a need for improved nutrition and socialization. Your Area Agency (or Council) on Aging should be able to provide information about these congregate dining sites.

PERSONAL CARE OR HOMEMAKER SERVICES

In most communities there are businesses or organizations that provide nonmedical care for individuals who need assistance with some of their everyday responsibilities and activities. These services enable individuals to remain in their own homes and continue with many of their routines and activities. Among the services offered by these organizations are meal preparation and cleanup, light housekeeping, laundry and ironing, changing linens, medication reminders, mailing bills and letters, assisting with pet care, grocery shopping, incidental transportation, and escorting to appointments, meetings, and religious services. In addition to compiling a list of these organizations in your community, congregations can sponsor programs at which representatives of these organizations discuss the services they offer.

HOME HEALTH CARE

Individuals who need certain types of health care but are homebound or normally unable to leave home unassisted may need the services of a home health agency. Home health agencies provide and help coordinate the care ordered by a physician. These organizations offer a range of skilled care services, including nursing care, physical and occupational therapy, speech-language therapy, and medical social services. Information about the home health agencies in your community and eligibility for Medicare coverage of these services is available at www.medicare.gov.

SUPPORT GROUPS

The challenges of living with the limitations and uncertainties of a chronic illness can leave the affected individuals, and sometime their caregivers, feeling overwhelmed, emotionally drained, and deeply discouraged about their long-term prospects. Support groups, in which people facing similar health concerns and challenges gather on a regular basis, give individuals an opportunity to share their feelings and learn how to cope with the most difficult aspects of their situation. Members often receive assistance with the practical as well as emotional aspects of their illnesses, learning new problem-solving strategies and discovering additional community resources.

Identifying the various support groups in most communities can be challenging. Although some hospitals and community agencies maintain a list of support groups, in many communities there is no comprehensive list. A good place to start your research into this matter is to visit the Web site of your local hospital or contact the hospital's case management or social work department to see if they have a list of support groups. If they do not have a list, you will need to use your telephone and the Internet to compile a list. You can start by visiting the Web sites of national organizations associated with specific conditions (e.g., Alzheimer's Association, American Stroke Association, American Cancer Society, Mental Health America). Many of these include contact information about support groups throughout the country or links to local chapters that have information about support groups. Another strategy is to call physicians' offices. For example, neurologists may be aware of support groups for those who have had a stroke or have Parkinson's disease, and oncologists may have information about cancer support groups.

FINANCIAL COUNSELING AND ASSISTANCE

For some individuals who have debilitating chronic illnesses, handling basic finances can be a problem. Although they may have adequate resources, they find it difficult to handle certain financial responsibilities. In some communities the Area Agency on Aging or another community agency can arrange for a financial care manager to assume these responsibilities—making deposits, writing checks to pay the client's bills, and balancing checkbooks and bank statements. Clients can still maintain the responsibility for directing which bills should be paid and signing the checks. Another option in many communities is to arrange for a bank to electronically pay bills from the customer's account. The customer or a family member can monitor the account via the bank's online service—checking account activity and balances, viewing statements online, viewing images of paid checks, and transferring funds between accounts. The congregational health ministry team can explore various options and publish a list of organizations that provide these services.

LEGAL ASSISTANCE

Affected individuals or their families may need to obtain legal assistance for a number of illness-related challenges. These include Medicare claims and appeals, disability claims and appeals, guardianships, and disability planning, including the use of durable power of attorney, living wills, and other means of delegating management and decision making in the case of incapacity. As with many issues, the best time to learn about these is well in advance of a crisis. It is helpful for a congregational health ministry team to identify local attorneys who have experience in these areas of law and invite them to speak at a seminar.

RESPITE CARE AND ADULT DAY CARE

For many individuals, their ability to remain in their own home depends largely on having a spouse or other family member live with them and provide much of their care. This arrangement often works well, but it can place considerable stress on caregivers, who may find they do not have enough time to take care of their own responsibilities or that the strain of caregiving is jeopardizing their own physical or mental health. When this occurs, caregivers can consider several options to relieve some of the stress. For those who are capable of providing most of the care for a loved one but need some time away to tend to their own responsibilities and needs, respite care can be a good option. Some respite care programs provide an in-home companion, while others have a facility where the person in need of care can stay for a few hours. In some communities, organizations serving older adults have partnered with religious congregations to offer respite programs. When family caregivers need to go out of town for a few days or require medical treatment that will temporarily prevent them from providing care, skilled nursing facilities may be able to provide respite care. When individuals with a debilitating chronic illness cannot be left alone but the family caregiver has full-time work responsibilities, adult day care centers that offer a protective and supportive setting may be the best alternative.

The congregational health ministry team can provide a valuable service by exploring respite care and adult day care services in the community. Your research can start by contacting the Area Agency on Aging or the case management or social work department of your local hospital, but it can also include visiting programs to evaluate their facilities and services. Some congregations may want to explore offering their facilities and providing volunteers for a respite care program one or two days a week; if so, it is advisable to work closely with experienced professionals (e.g., hospital administrators, Area Agency on Aging staff) to ensure that the facilities meet any applicable regulatory and licensing requirements, the environment is safe, and volunteers are properly trained and supervised.

CARE MANAGEMENT

For some individuals with chronic illnesses, the extent of their impairment and the services they require to live independently are not readily apparent. In such cases, the services of a care manager may be helpful. Geriatric care managers are health or human services professionals who can assess an individual's medical and human service needs and then assist in making arrangements for the provision of the required services. Care managers also can make regular visits to monitor the care and status of their client, determining if any new challenges have arisen and additional services should be considered. Should the time come that the client is no longer able to live independently, the care manager can assist in finding the most appropriate living arrangement. The services of a care manager can be especially helpful when the family members who have assumed responsibility for the care of a loved one live in a distant community. To identify geriatric care managers in your community, you can contact your local Area Agency on Aging or visit the Web site for the National Association of Professional Geriatric Care Managers (www.napgcm.org).

LONG-TERM CARE RESOURCES

There may come a time when individuals find that they are no longer able to live independently or that their quality of life will be better if they move to a community or facility that can provide more comprehensive care and greater security. A congregational health ministry team can assist these individuals and their families by compiling a list of the various housing options in the community and providing information about their services, costs, and eligibility requirements. Four long-term care options are available in most communities.

Continuing Care Retirement Community (CCRC) or Life Care Community. These communities combine independent living, assisted living, and skilled nursing care in one setting. Individuals can start off living independently in their own apartment, townhouse, or cottage and then add services (e.g., meals, housekeeping, and transportation) or transfer to an on-site assisted living or skilled nursing care facility as their needs change. Many of these communities offer primary and preventive health care services. Residents generally pay an entry fee and then monthly maintenance fees. Entry fees, policies on refunds of entry fees, monthly maintenance fees, and fees for additional services and amenities vary widely.

Assisted Living Facility (ALF) or Adult Congregate Living Care. These facilities are generally appropriate for individuals who need assistance with activities of daily living but do not require skilled nursing care. The types of service and levels of care can vary, but assisted living facilities typically provide assistance with bathing, dressing, eating, and monitoring of medications. Meals, laundry, and housekeeping are also provided, and some facilities arrange for transportation and offer regular social programs and activities. Residents generally pay a monthly rental fee that covers most of the basic services. Additional fees may be required for certain services.

Skilled Nursing Facility or Nursing Home. These facilities are appropriate for individuals who require skilled medical care. Although some may need to be in this setting only on a temporary basis while rehabilitating from an illness or injury, others may spend the rest of their lives in this setting due to physical, cognitive, or emotional conditions that require ongoing medical and personal care. Skilled nursing facilities provide a room (private or shared), all meals, 24-hour nursing supervision, access to needed medical services, personal care, and generally some social activities. A physician supervises the medical care of residents. Some nursing homes provide additional services for a fee.

Hospice. Hospice care is appropriate when the goal of an individual with a terminal illness has shifted from cure or life-prolonging treatment to palliative care (i.e., care aimed at relieving pain and controlling symptoms). Most hospices accept patients who have a life expectancy of six months or less if their disease runs its normal course (the requirement for Medicare reimbursement), although some are able to accept patients with a longer life expectancy. Hospice care is provided by a team that includes doctors, nurses, social workers, chaplains, pharmacists, home health aides, and volunteers, and this care can be provided in a person's home, in a nursing home, or in a residential care center.

Hospice services continue to be underused, with many eligible individuals never using hospice care and others electing it only in their final few days or weeks of life. At least some of this under-use is the result of misunderstandings about hospice care. Some people believe it is only for individuals who have cancer or AIDS, and others assume it is appropriate only when death is imminent. Hospice is often appropriate for individuals who have conditions such as advanced emphysema, heart failure, or dementia. Congregational health ministry teams can perform an important service by educating their congregations and communities about the nature of hospice care, the medical conditions for which it might be appropriate, and the point at which individuals and families may want to consider electing hospice care.

EXAMPLE OF A CONGREGATIONAL PROGRAM

An example of how representatives of faith communities can work with medical institutions and professionals to help individuals identify and access community resources is the ElderCare Project, a care transition program provided to patients by volunteer parish nurses associated with the Sacred Heart Health System (a part of Ascension Health in Pensacola, Florida). Much of the program's structure was taken from the "nurse coach" model developed through the work of Dr. Eric Coleman of the University of Colorado. The ElderCare program is funded by donations from the Escambia County Medical Society, with additional funds and in-kind services provided by a number of civic groups, health care services, and private individuals.

The mission of the ElderCare Project is to link at-risk seniors who do not have a capable caregiver living with them to appropriate health and social services, thus allowing them to live independently in their own homes. Usually two nurses make the initial home visit and do an in-depth assessment of the patient's health status and needs. Once the assessment is completed, identified needs are conveyed to a case manager at the Council on Aging or to a community agency that may be able to assist. If the nurses find a medical issue that needs to be addressed before the patient's next medical appointment, they contact (with the patient's approval) the physician or the on-call nurse practitioner who volunteers with the ElderCare project. Medication issues are managed in a number of different ways, including consulting with volunteer pharmacists from a local Veterans Administration (VA) clinic. After the initial face-to-face visit, the nurses arrange for follow-up phone calls with the patient to ensure that health and social service needs are being met.

Cheryl Pilling, M.A., B.S.N., the coordinator for Community Wellness Outreach and ElderCare Health at Sacred Heart Health System, offers the following case as an illustration of how the program operates.

A woman in her late seventies had been placed on a new blood pressure medication by her primary care physician during her hospitalization. Because of her ongoing weakness and memory problems, she was directed not to drive. Up to several months before her hospitalization, she had been essentially self-sufficient. Now she had to depend on her two children, one who lived about

twenty miles away and the other who was legally blind, to assist her. Two par-
ish nurses, acting as ElderCare nurse coaches, made their home visit and dis-
covered that this patient needed home-delivered meals because she had diffi-
culty standing to cook, had missed her follow-up doctor's appointment, was
out of the new blood pressure medication, and did not know what to do.

Thanks to the parish nurses' interventions, the physician's office sent a
physician's assistant to the patient's home, who brought more medication,
determined that she needed more assistance, and ordered home care. She was
also able to obtain meals delivered to her home, a service that reduced her
anxiety over not being able to get out and purchase groceries and cook for
herself. And having the physician's assistant make home visits meant that she
would not miss any more doctor's appointments.

INFORMATION RESOURCES

Information and advice on housing options and links to additional resources can be found at www.aoa.dhhs.gov/eldfam/Housing/Housing.asp (the Web site for the Administration on Aging). The AARP Web site (www.aarp.org) also provides information on housing options.

17

INNOVATIVE MEDICAL-RELIGIOUS PARTNERSHIPS

The health needs and concerns that can be addressed by medical-religious partnerships vary from community to community. This chapter presents five different programs. Our own report on a program serving Daytona Beach and surrounding communities is followed by a report on a program in Memphis (prepared by Gary Gunderson), information on several programs offered in communities served by Ascension Health (prepared by Fran Zoske), a description of a program based in south Florida (prepared by Dale Young), and a report on a program serving the greater Orlando area (prepared by Candace Huber).

THE O'NEILL FOUNDATION FOR COMMUNITY HEALTH

The O'Neill Foundation for Community Health, a tax-exempt, non-profit organization, works with religious congregations, health care organizations, social service agencies, and educational institutions throughout the United States to provide the resources people need to maintain their own health and to care for sick or disabled individuals. The foundation's goals are:

- To provide training programs and ongoing support for clergy and members of religious congregations who are interested in developing health ministries
- To produce educational materials and other resources that clergy,

parish/faith community nurses, and volunteer health ministry coordinators can use to address the health needs of their congregations and communities

• To facilitate collaboration between religious institutions and medical organizations

The O'Neill Foundation traces its roots back to 1992, when the authors collaborated in the development of a curriculum used to train volunteers from faith communities to coordinate health programs. Volunteers were taught how to organize programs on a wide range of conditions and medical issues, including Alzheimer's disease, heart disease, hypertension, cancer, depression, diabetes, managing medications, advance directives, and preventing accidents. Hospitals and medical professionals participated, collaborating with volunteers to conduct health education programs, screenings, and preventive interventions in their congregations. Building on the success of these programs and in response to needs of many of the older adults with whom we worked, we subsequently developed a program to train volunteers to serve as patient advocates or health partners for individuals who do not have a relative or friend to accompany them to doctor visits or help coordinate various aspects of their care.

Interest in these programs exceeded our initial expectations. The workshops attracted volunteers eager to learn more about important medical issues and how they could organize health programs for their congregations and, in many cases, for the community at large. As word of the programs spread, more congregations became involved, and so did more hospitals and health care professionals. It was clear that these programs were meeting an important need.

Critical to the success of these programs was the support of Mr. and Mrs. William E. O'Neill, of Daytona Beach, Florida. Longtime supporters of religious, medical, and educational institutions, they recognized the potential of programs that harnessed the energy of committed members of faith communities and coupled it with information and resources provided by health care professionals. In 2003 the O'Neills offered to establish a charitable foundation to provide ongoing support for this effort.

The O'Neill Foundation is headquartered in Volusia County, Florida, which serves as an ideal "field laboratory" for developing and evaluating new programs because the county has a sizable population of older adults.

In fact, the proportion of the population age 65 or older—20 percent—is the same as that projected for the entire United States by 2030.

One of the first steps the O'Neill Foundation took as part of an effort to develop an innovative faith-health initiative was to compile a list of all religious congregations in the county. We found nearly five hundred faith communities in this county of approximately 500,000 people. A letter introducing the foundation and its plans was sent to each of these congregations, and those that were not interested in receiving further information could opt to have their name removed from the mailing list. Only five congregations asked that we do this.

The foundation then contacted each of the seven hospitals in the county (Bert Fish Medical Center in New Smyrna Beach, Florida Hospital DeLand, Florida Hospital Fish Memorial in Orange City, Florida Hospital Oceanside in Daytona Beach, Florida Hospital Ormond Memorial in Ormond Beach, Halifax Health Medical Center in Daytona Beach, and Halifax Health Port Orange) to invite them to serve as partners with the foundation. All seven accepted the invitation and offered financial support and assistance in planning and promoting health education programs. Also joining as partners were the Volusia County Health Department, the Council on Aging, the Hospice of Volusia/Flagler, Stetson University, and Bethune-Cookman University.

Each year the foundation, in consultation with its partners, selects several timely health topics to serve as the focus of a Congregational and Community Health Initiative. As part of this initiative, the foundation produces materials, including taped interviews with medical experts from the Johns Hopkins Medical Institutions designed specifically for faith communities. The format of these materials is such that they can be used to organize special congregational programs, presented during regularly scheduled congregational gatherings or taken home and viewed by individual members. Topics include Alzheimer's disease, depression, diabetes, cancer, heart disease, palliative care, chronic disease in African Americans, and making the most of a medical visit.

As part of its annual Congregational and Community Health Initiative, the foundation and its partners sponsor one or more major conferences on medical topics that have been found to be of concern to the community. Although the conferences are open to the entire community, special invitations are sent to all religious congregations, and speakers include in their presentations suggestions for how congregations can address some of the needs associated with the medical issues being discussed. The foundation also tapes the presentations and makes these available on DVD at no charge to individuals who are unable to attend and to those who do attend and wish to share the information with other individuals or groups.

An example of the foundation's multifaceted community health initiatives is one that focused on Alzheimer's disease in the fall of 2007. The centerpiece of this program consisted of two presentations (one on each side of the county) on "Alzheimer's Disease: Challenges for Professionals and Caregivers" by Dr. Peter Rabins, a geriatric psychiatrist on the faculty at the Johns Hopkins University School of Medicine and co-author of the best-selling book, *The 36-Hour Day: A Family Guide to Caring for People with Alzheimer Disease, Other Dementias, and Memory Loss in Later Life.* The hospitals and other organizations that serve as the O'Neill Foundation's partners co-sponsored the event, with each organization sharing information about its services and programs. But these presentations were only part of a comprehensive initiative to reach out into the community. The first part of this initiative had come a month earlier when the foundation mailed to each of the congregations on its mailing list not only an invitation to send representatives to attend one of Dr. Rabins's presentations but also a copy of his book that could be placed in the congregation's office or library for use by anyone who needed information on Alzheimer's disease.

The third part of the foundation's initiative involved videotaping one of Dr. Rabins's presentations and then making copies of the DVD available at no charge to anyone who believed that he or she knew other individuals or groups who would benefit from the information. Of the more than 700 people who attended this conference, 250 requested a copy of the DVD. Individuals requesting a copy were asked to estimate the number of people who would view the tape over the next twelve months; the estimates totaled more than 9,000.

A similar community health initiative, this one focusing on "Recognizing and Responding to Depression" and again featuring Dr. Peter Rabins as the guest speaker, was organized by the foundation in the spring of 2008. This time the foundation mailed to all religious congregations in the county an invitation to hear Dr. Rabins and a 24-page booklet on depression prepared by the National Institute of Mental Health. The foundation also arranged to have one of Dr. Rabins's presentations videotaped and copies of the presentation made available to individuals who heard the presentation and knew of others who would benefit from the information. Of the more than 600 people who attended one of Dr. Rabins's presentations, 210 requested a copy, and their estimates of the number of people who would see the video over the next twelve months totaled almost 5,000.

In addition to these major, high-visibility initiatives, the foundation co-sponsors with individual hospitals a number of smaller programs targeting congregations near each hospital. Among the topics covered in these programs are accident and fall prevention, advance directives, modifying risk factors for cardiovascular disease and diabetes, stress management, and hospice and palliative care. The foundation stays in touch with local congregations by mailing newsletters and maintaining a Web site, with both providing information about timely health topics and local health resources. Bulletin inserts with information about health programs and services are also mailed to congregations.

The foundation conducts workshops for clergy and laypersons interested in establishing health ministries or expanding existing programs. No medical experience or background is required to enroll in these workshops, just a strong interest in serving others and good organizational skills. The workshops are often co-sponsored by religious, medical, or educational institutions.

The O'Neill Foundation offers consultation services and workshops for health care organizations interested in developing partnerships with or educational programs for faith communities. More information about programs and materials can be obtained by contacting the foundation or visiting its Web site: O'Neill Foundation for Community Health, P.O. Box 1529, DeLand, FL 32721-1529; (386) 748-3775; www.oneillcommunityhealth.org.

THE CONGREGATIONAL HEALTH NETWORK OF MEMPHIS, TENNESSEE

Memphis is a tough town with a bitter legacy of health disparities that appear to many to be intractable. Some of the downtown neighborhoods have infant mortality rates comparable to those in Zimbabwe, while rates of poorly managed and early-onset chronic disease are epidemic. One might expect faith-based health projects to be modest, perhaps focused on devising pilot approaches that could be scaled up later. But this is the ground where the dream of Dr. King's "beloved community" continues to thrive forty years after its dreamer was killed. It is a city where dreams don't die.

The Congregational Health Network (CHN) is a young but significant network of 105 churches and Methodist LeBonheur Healthcare that have entered into a covenant with each other to share the ministry of improving the health of members and neighbors. The covenant is focused on helping people navigate their journey of life, which will probably, from time to time, involve some aspect of the medical system, even a hospital. Hospital research indicates that 70 percent of emergency room patients in Memphis have been in a house of worship within the last 30 days, indicating that the congregation is the critical care network of the majority of patients before they enter into a medical care environment. As Gary Shorb, the CEO of Methodist LeBonheur Healthcare, says, "We want to connect the faith-based treatment system (us) with the faith-based health system (the congregations)." The current 105 congregations signed up within the first nine months of the program. Expectations are that, within a couple of years, 20 percent of the more than 2,000 congregations within an hour or so of downtown—roughly 400—will enter the covenant.

The covenant provides the logic of the infrastructure that is emerging in the shared space between hospital and congregation. Both already have extensive infrastructure; only the web of relationship between them is new. That scaffolding includes a full-time "navigator" at each hospital whose primary job is to know and build the caring capacity of the congregations closest to that facility. Each pastor appoints at least one "liaison" whose job is to build the caring pathway with the navigator. Thinking of it as scaffolding emphasizes that it is under construction, because the pathway differs depending on the nature, size, capacity, and demographics of each congregation. The navigators are trained to appreciate the strengths the congregations already have and then to follow the intelligence of its clergy and laypeople about where best to extend those strengths.

The hospital does not prescribe any particular program: some of the congregations have Stephen Ministers (laypersons trained to provide one-to-one Christian care; see www.stephenministries.org for more information); others have parish nurses or lay health workers; some are just now organizing a health committee. The hospital offers specific training related to spiritual care visitation that is designed to build the confidence and competence of laity and clergy to share the spiritual care of their members and neighbors when in the hospital. The seven-week classes are limited to 40 participants and tend to fill up months in advance. About half of the graduates volunteer to share the care of the general inpatient population beyond their own members.

The evidence base on which the Congregational Health Network rests is not programmatic, but social. This reflects the often-overlooked work of Ellen Idler of Rutgers University, which strongly suggests that the positive effect of congregational participation on peoples' lifespan is achieved at low levels of technical sophistication. The "intervention" is the whole thing: the complex, unpredictably relevant social support and engagement that happens in a congregation. CHN focuses on the existing social network of the congregation and its neighborhood, not on any particular added program. The health programs of various sorts add powerfully to the underlying social strengths a congregation already expresses without ever noticing that it is doing "health ministry." This perspective reflects the eight congregational strengths of *Deeply Woven Roots* (Gunderson 1997), but those strengths would exist regardless of the book.

The work in Memphis adapts the work of the African Religious Health Assets Programme (ARHAP) based at the University of Cape Town, South Africa. Using a blend of geographical information system mapping, participatory appreciative inquiry, and qualitative social science, ARHAP has shown how to see what is on the ground in Memphis that contributes to the health of the city. Although the hospital has hundreds of millions of dollars and most congregations do not, the most powerful health assets lie in the congregations, even the tiny ones led by clergy who have no formal seminary training. The art and, Idler would say, science, is in how to align the health assets of all sectors so that the journey of life reflects what God has in mind. That alignment begins with a covenant built on shared humility that is just as curious about what the hospital knows about congregational vitality as it is about what the congregation knows about health.

This humility is visible in the heart of the covenant, a document that emerged from a mixture of clergy and health system intelligence.

Methodist Le Bonheur Healthcare (Hospital System) agrees to:
Extend to partnering clergy the following benefits already extended to United Methodist clergy:

- Admission to clergy wellness events and programs
- Up to a 60 percent discount off the total Methodist LeBonheur Healthcare charges (not to exceed the balance after payment by your insurance)
- Tuition waiver to Methodist LeBonheur Healthcare clinical pastoral education
- Health-related training experiences, made available and affordable to partner clergy through work with local and national academic partners

To share in the work of aligning the mutual strengths of congregation and health system, we will:

- Provide a dedicated hospital navigator assigned to work with partner congregations to coordinate and help train members on the partnership activities with the congregation
- Work with expert partners such as the Church Health Center and Memphis Theological Seminary to help assess, plan, and build the education, prevention, intervention, treatment, and aftercare support that will be appropriate to the partnership congregations
- Provide ongoing support, training, and appropriate resources for the partnership with the partner clergy
- Partner to monitor, review, and expand the Congregational Health Network (CHN)

Clergy agree to:

- Attend quarterly clergy partnership gatherings for mutual training, awareness, and encouragement
- Provide ongoing leadership to monitor, review, and expand the CHN
- Use the clergy role to articulate and mirror the values and practices of a healthy lifestyle
- Extend an opportunity for members/neighbors to be informed of the program and benefits and to become active participants
- Provide leadership training for an active health ministry in the congregation. This group will be involved in education/prevention for members and neighbors. They will also have a role in intervention/aftercare if a member or neighbor is hospitalized.
- Assign a congregational liaison to facilitate the program
- Seek ways to help other clergy, health system staff, and congregations pursue healthy lifestyles and common goals

- Continue to support the partnership in prayer and worship to become God's instruments for health and wholeness in our community

Congregational Health Network is not owned by the hospital or by any one of the congregations. It is emerging through a kind of co-creation that in itself is healthy and builds the confidence and strength of all the partners. The future will emerge through the continued work of paying close attention to the real journeys the members and neighbors are taking. It offers individual members the opportunity to register through their congregation so that they have an ID card and are entered into the Methodist LeBonheur Healthcare's electronic medical record system. This allows CHN to activate the congregational support network just as with other parts of the care technology environment. The system also enables CHN to engage in "back-end data capture" to track health outcomes by comparing CHN members' health status (e.g., average length of stay) to those of non-CHN peers over time. CHN members' health status, ultimately, may demonstrate the capacity and vitality of CHN webs of trust to move Memphis toward the Beloved Community envisioned by Dr. King more than forty years ago.

For more information on the Congregational Health Network of Memphis, contact Teresa Cutts, Director of Research and Praxis, Center of Excellence in Faith and Health, Methodist LeBonheur Healthcare, 1211 Union Avenue, Memphis, Tennessee 38104, cutts02@gmail.com.

ASCENSION HEALTH

Ascension Health was founded in 1999 and today is the largest Catholic and largest nonprofit health system in the United States. It was formed through the merger of two health care systems, the Daughters of Charity Health System and the Congregation of the Sisters of St. Joseph's. The Daughters of Charity National Health System included nearly 80 facilities in 15 states, and the Sisters of St. Joseph Health System had four regional systems operating more than 30 hospitals, nursing homes, and outpatient clinics throughout lower Michigan. In 2002 the Sisters of St. Joseph of Carondelet joined, adding 13 more health care institutions to the Ascension system. Since that time, Ascension Health has achieved recognition as a model of leadership and clinical excellence in U.S. health care.

The Ascension Health ministry is dedicated to spiritually centered, holistic care that sustains and improves the health of individuals and communities. It is not surprising, then, that faith community nursing (also known as parish nursing) has long been a part not only of Ascension Health but also of the founding organizations. The values and goals of this system—service to the poor, reverence, and integrity—provide the spiritual foundation for Ascension Health's faith community nurses. The faith community nurses view themselves as advocates for a compassionate and just society.

The faith community nursing movement within Ascension Health can be traced back through its founding organizations, with the first programs beginning in 1986 at Seton Health of Troy, New York (a Daughters of Charity–sponsored health system), and in 1989 at St. John Health of Warren, Michigan (a Sisters of St. Joseph's–sponsored health system). Today more than a thousand nurses function in the role of faith community nurse within Ascension Health, making this the largest cohort of faith community nurses in one national health care system.

The Ascension Health Faith Community Nurse Leadership Network was founded in 2004 with the acknowledgment by Ascension Health of the importance of this growing nursing specialty. A Web site was instrumental in breaking down the barriers brought on by distance. The Ascension Exchange Faith Community Nurses Web site allowed individual members to seek out common endeavors, identify best practices, and address on a national level specific health issues common to all. One significant event solidified this group: this new network provided important feedback to the Health Ministries Association and the American Nurses Association in the revision of *Faith Community Nursing: Scope and Standards of Practice* (2005). In 2006, Ascension Health gave financial support to the University of Albany to conduct a survey of this network that would become the first enumeration study of faith community nurses in the United States. The current network includes faith community nursing leaders representing 22 health systems within Ascension Health.

The strategic priorities of Ascension Health's faith community nurses can be found at the local and national levels. Some initiatives are best addressed by local leaders within the context of the community needs; others require collaborative engagement as a national ministry. Their stories illustrate the many ways in which these faith community nurses have facilitated and/or improved clinical excellence and safety; created innovative, patient-centered environments; and expanded access to care for uninsured and underserved individuals.

At Borgess Health in Kalamazoo, Michigan, faith community nurses reach out to their community with emphasis on spiritual beliefs and practices. Individuals identified by parish staff or by self-referral receive home visits by the faith community nurse and pastor that allow for an assessment of individual needs, resources currently being used, and additional resources that are needed. These visits include prayer; information gathering; problem solving; and referrals to appropriate parish, community, and health care resources. The faith community nurse and pastor then determine the type of follow-up needed and coordinate their contacts with the individual.

The Borgess Health nurses collect, analyze, prioritize, and document comprehensive data pertinent to the holistic health of individuals in the community. Faith community nurses, in collaboration with health cabinets and pastoral staff, conduct a health survey of the congregation within the first year of ministry and periodically thereafter. Results are aggregated, analyzed, reported to congregational leadership, and used in planning health ministry activities. They also recruit, train, and support volunteers and identify strengths that enhance the health and spiritual well-being of others.

Faith community nurses at Borgess Health identified a lack of support for pregnant, non-English-speaking Hispanic women. The Mother-Friend program was developed through a collaborative relationship among community agencies, area churches, and OB professionals to provide bilingual volunteers to mentor and support women in need through the pregnancy and the baby's first year of life. Mother-Friends are given an orientation to their role and information about prenatal care routines; current labor, delivery, and infant care practices; and postnatal care needs. They are offered ongoing in-service education and support through a Mother-Friend program at a local agency as they mentor young mothers.

At Seton Health, in Troy, New York, faith community nurses reaching out to diverse communities used evidence-based practices and assessment techniques to address adolescent obesity within an African American community. Recognizing the effect obesity was having on the children within their community, faith community nurses at Bethel Baptist Church, an African American church in Troy, obtained a local grant to develop an aerobic exercise program for teens. The program, Pray Hard and Move Your Feet, was held on a weekly basis, led by a certified aerobic instructor using hip hop music. As the children were dancing, parents were invited to attend a cooking lesson given by a diabetes educator with the purpose of teaching healthier eating choices.

Reyut's Faith Community Nursing Program, a committee of the Women's Network of Congregation Agudat Achim (a Jewish synagogue in Schenectady, New York, and a member of the Seton Health Faith Community Nursing Network), supports members of their congregation through life's transitions while they grow spiritually and remain an integral part of the Jewish community. Reyut (a Hebrew word meaning "friendship") is working to create a caring congregation and is composed of volunteers who provide transportation to the synagogue, the doctor's office, or other activities. The volunteers also visit homebound members, hospitalized members, and members residing in nursing homes. Educational presentations focusing on health promotion, illness prevention, and caregivers' issues are offered on a monthly basis.

M.O.S.T. (Men of St. Timothy's Lutheran Church in East Greenbush, NY) began when the faith community nurse identified numerous health concerns voiced by male members of the church on the health needs survey. Using the services of a men's health consultant, a focus group was held with male members of the congregation. The men requested an ongoing support and spiritual group. The group, using the Carpenters Bible, was able to identify and address various physical, emotional, and spiritual concerns of male members and went on to hold yearly father-son breakfasts on Father's Day, bringing in guest speakers to discuss these issues.

In 2002–2003, at St. Agnes of Baltimore, Maryland, faith community nurses obtained a grant from Kaiser Permanente for the Faith Community Diabetes Self-Management Project. Training was provided to congregational health ministry leaders who facilitated monthly meetings for groups of ten members diagnosed with diabetes, using American Diabetes Association guidelines. Data were collected on seven diabetes education outcome areas. Participants reported a 10–20 percent increase in all data points: knowledge, skills, and confidence.

At Genesys Health System, of Grand Blanc, Michigan, faith community nurses strengthen and enhance health and spiritual well-being through advocacy. A faith community nurse worked with a mother of a severely disabled 12-year-old, advocating for resources that would allow the child to remain in her home under her mother's care. The nurse helped reaffirm the mother's strengths, and this assistance has helped to keep the family together.

The Genesys nurses also serve as referral agents. During a blood pressure screening, a man became faint and pale and had a low blood pressure reading. The parish nurse provided him with a copy of the reading and encouraged him to call his physician. He made an appointment with the physician for follow-up and further exploration of signs and symptoms.

At Lourdes Hospital, in Binghamton, New York, faith community nurses reached out to the larger community by providing blood pressure screenings at the local soup kitchen and health fairs in various counties of the Southern Tier area of New York. They also addressed the needs of uninsured and underinsured individuals by bringing resources to area faith communities during Access to Care month. Individuals in need of insurance could speak to local insurance companies as well as to Child Health Plus representatives and sign up for health insurance.

At St. Vincent Medical Center in Bridgeport, Connecticut, the faith community nursing program is a valuable health information resource center. It provides weekly health talks in parishes, health tips in Sunday bulletins, a caregivers resource and nursing home placement guide, a speakers bureau guide to various community agencies, and a guide on medications with information on potential side effects and possible interactions with over-the-counter medicines.

For more information on Ascension Health, contact Fran Zoske, M.S., R.N., FCN, Director, Health Promotion and Wellness, CDPHP, 500 Patroon Creek Blvd., Albany, NY 12206-1057, fzoske@cdphp.com.

CONGREGATIONAL HEALTH ALLIANCE
MINISTRY PROGRAM

In 1986, after evaluating the changes and impact of managed care on health, Baptist Health South Florida, the region's largest not-for-profit health care organization, formed an advisory board to create a partnership between the health system and area faith communities. The advisory board, made up of professionals in the health system as well as clergy and volunteers from the community, modified the "parish nurse model" of the Midwest to suit the social-economic-cultural context of the Miami area. This new model, the Congregational Health Alliance Ministry Program (CHAMP), trains volunteer community health promoters to develop congregation-based health ministries.

Three trends in health care created the contextual situation that the CHAMP model addressed:

1. Numerous research studies showed that patients who receive religious support and are connected to their faith or their religious community experience better health outcomes than patients who are not connected to their faith or their religious community. Doctors, nurses, social workers, and, most important, health care administrators paid attention to the research and began asking for more spiritual/religious support for hospitalized patients.

2. Managed care resulted in a significant reduction in the number of days patients stayed in the hospital and an increase in the number of outpatient surgeries. This meant that patients would be receiving less spiritual support in the hospital and would have a greater need for support by the faith communities following discharge. The change in context required a shift from providing institution-based spiritual support toward congregation-based support.

3. The tourist and agricultural-based economy of south Florida tends to create jobs that do not provide health insurance. Some 600,000 area residents lack health insurance. Additionally, new immigrants, especially if undocumented, tend to be marginalized with respect to health care delivery systems. The poor, the uninsured, new immigrants, and part-time workers have two things in common: they lack preventive care measures such as health education and screenings, and they have less access to health care.

The need for health promotion in the community became increasingly evident. CHAMP began to build capacity in the faith community to respond to these changing trends.

The CHAMP mission is to develop and strengthen a network of health ministries in faith communities. CHAMP promotes congregation-based programs of health education, health screenings, home visitation of sick people, bereavement support, care teams, and practical/spiritual support to individuals with health challenges. CHAMP has trained, assisted, and supported more than 85 area congregations that currently network to promote health in the community.

The CHAMP model envisioned a two-prong strategy to meet the contemporary challenges: health promotion and support of the sick.

In the first part of the strategy, building capacity in the faith communities took the form of health education, health promotion, and health screenings based on specific "congregational health profiles." Each congregation in the CHAMP network designed its own health promotion program based on the results of a congregational health profile. Programs developed in this strategy include: health education events, health fairs, health screenings, and health support groups. In 2007, CHAMP offered free health screenings (e.g., blood sugar, cholesterol, osteoporosis, etc.) at 26 congregational health fairs. Since 1999, more than 22,700 free health screenings have been done through the CHAMP network.

The second part of the strategy focuses on support of those who have health challenges and are at home. There are three components to this facet of the CHAMP model: faith-based health support groups, care teams, and bereavement support.

Faith-Based Health Support Groups

Faith-based health support groups function within the life of the partnering congregations and focus on specific health issues (cancer, diabetes, depression, Alzheimer's disease, etc.). Through these peer support health promotion groups, congregations are becoming agents of healing and wholeness. CHAMP has established working partnerships with health promotion organizations such as the American Heart Association, the American Diabetes Association, the local chapter of the National Alliance on Mental Illness, the Alzheimer's Association of South Florida, and the Alliance for Aging. For example, when CHAMP trains leaders for health support groups with a healthy heart focus, it invites the American Heart Association to participate in the training and the follow-up support, using the materials that AHA developed for use in faith communities.

Congregation-Based Care Teams

Congregation-based care teams are designed to meet the challenges of patients recovering at home following hospitalization. Before designing the care teams model, CHAMP conducted a focus group of seniors to learn about the gaps in services they experienced after a period of hospitalization. Even among those who had good health insurance, there were many gaps in care and many needs that health care providers and community organizations were not able to meet: transportation to the doctor for follow-up visits, transportation to purchase prescriptions and food, meal preparation, light housekeeping, errands, companioning, caregiver relief, and spiritual support. CHAMP designed the care teams model to fill the gaps identified by the seniors.

To successfully implement the care teams model, CHAMP developed a curriculum to train volunteers to do holistic assessments and to organize and administer a care teams program in their respective congregations. A training course was developed to build capacity within partnering congregations and to train, enable, and support congregation-based care team programs. "Post-Hospitalization Spiritual Care" is a 32-hour curriculum that includes holistic patient assessment, spiritual assessment, self-care, active listening, infection control, advance directives, confidentiality, organizational model, and administration of a care teams program. While doing this work, CHAMP learned that the staff needed to focus on the spirituality of aging and the spiritual challenges implicit in facing end-of-life decisions. Those and other emerging issues were incorporated into the training course. CHAMP also learned that volunteers who served on care teams found it a meaningful activity. One of the volunteers stated, "If I could do this full time, I'd quit my regular job and do this every day."

Once a team from a congregation is trained, they organize care teams and set the parameters of the program in their respective congregation. To solidify the link between the hospitals and the faith community care teams, CHAMP established a procedure to make referrals from the hospital. CHAMP consulted with chaplains, social workers, and discharge planners before creating a guide that would facilitate the referral of patients to the faith-based care teams. Using this referral guide, discharge planners, social workers, and chaplains may easily refer a patient to an appropriate care team. Congregational membership, language, culture, and location are factors in making referrals.

Eleven congregations have implemented the care team model and currently receive referrals from the chaplains and social workers of the Baptist Health system. By mid-2007 the CHAMP care teams had provided spiritual and practical support to more than 2,500 individuals. More than 200 congregational volunteers are involved in this ministry.

Services offered by partnering care teams include:

Meals delivered to the home
Transportation to medical appointments
Errands such as picking up medications and groceries
Home visitation and companioning
Caregiver relief
Light housekeeping
Spiritual support
Keep-in-touch phone contact

Bereavement Support

The CHAMP bereavement program received one of seven nation-wide grants from the Open Society Institute's Death in America Project in 2000. The objective of the grant was to establish a multicultural and cross-denominational grief support program in the faith community of Miami-Dade. There were three concerns in developing that program: (1) the desire to integrate spirituality into the bereavement support process; (2) the concern to integrate the wisdom and inherent cultural skills of Miami's diverse faith and cultural traditions; and (3) the goal to equip faith communities with professionally endorsed understanding of grief, empowering indigenous leadership to provide culturally appropriate peer group grief support. To date, CHAMP has trained more than 180 facilitators of bereavement support in Miami-Dade and the Upper Keys. CHAMP was invited to introduce this program in India and Sri Lanka following the Christmas Day 2005 Tsunami. In 2006 and 2007, more than 70 peer group grief support leaders in Sri Lanka and India were trained in the CHAMP bereavement support model.

The story of Susan illustrates how the CHAMP program works:

Susan came to Miami from New York to take care of her sister, Maryann, who was dying of cancer. Maryann was the caregiver of their brother, Michael, who had cerebral palsy. After Maryann died, Susan and Michael sought out one of the CHAMP bereavement programs, the network of peer group grief support programs in faith communities. They still attend after five years. Now, having worked through their own grief issues, they go to support others with their grief.

A few months ago, Susan had intestinal surgery and was hospitalized five days. She was discharged and that same evening was back in the ER with a blockage that required additional surgery. This time she stayed 14 days in the hospital. Once discharged, she had no one to help her. Her brother, who is on disability, cannot cook, cannot drive, and is basically dependent on Susan, who was in bed recovering. A friend went grocery shopping for her but then had to go out of town, and Susan was left with no help. She needed to go to five different doctors, needed medications, and could not even get out of bed.

Then she remembered about the CHAMP care teams program, so she called her church and got the number for the CHAMP office. Two churches in her Zip code had care team programs. A lady from the first church took her to the doctor, but Susan needed more support than that church could provide, so a second church got the referral. This church has more than 80 volunteers in the care teams program, and they went into action. The leader of the transportation team helped Susan organize her doctor visits and provided rides to her appointments, followed by trips to the pharmacy. They ran errands such as picking up prescriptions at the pharmacy and purchasing ready-to-eat meals and groceries. When Susan had a doctor's appointment, they would call the day before and also before picking her up, just to remind her. They provided care for a month and half.

When Susan was well enough to function on her own, the leader of the phone follow-up team would call once a week to see how she was doing. One month later, Susan became very sick. She called the doctor, and he prescribed medicine, but Susan had no way to pick up the medicine. She was desperate; she had no one she could call. Just then, there was a knock on the door and it was a lady from the CHAMP care team who had shown up just to see how she was doing. "It was like an angel had appeared," Susan said. She explained her predicament, and the visitor went to the pharmacy for her medicine.

Susan now tells everyone who will listen how wonderful are the ladies from the care teams and how she couldn't have made it without their support. Her own church is now organizing a care teams ministry, and Susan cannot wait to volunteer.

For more information about the CHAMP faith/health partnership, call 786-573-6087 or visit the Web site, www.baptisthealth.net/champ.

FLORIDA HOSPITAL'S PARISH NURSE INSTITUTE AND CENTER FOR COMMUNITY HEALTH MINISTRY

Florida Hospital is a not-for-profit, acute care health system with facilities in seven locations in the greater Orlando area. With more than 1,900 beds, it is the largest health system in the region. Florida Hospital is part of a comprehensive network of 17 hospitals of the Adventist Health System–Florida Division.

For nearly one hundred years, the stated mission of Florida Hospital has been "to extend the healing ministry of Jesus Christ." Adventist hospitals, inspired by the strong Adventist heritage of health ministry, work toward this goal through a commitment to patients' physical, mental, emotional, and spiritual well-being. This means that, in addition to treating illnesses, an important part of Florida Hospital's mission is to provide the support and education people need to prevent diseases and to live life to the fullest extent possible. The commitment to whole-person health is illustrated by CREATION Health, an acronym for the eight essentials of optimal health: Choice, Rest, Environment, Activity, Trust in divine power, Interpersonal relationships, Outlook, Nutrition. This commitment has inspired joint endeavors between the hospital and like-minded community resources.

Florida Hospital's Parish Nurse Institute was established in 1994. The following year, working in association with Stetson University, the hospital began offering the Lay Health Education Class developed by the authors, Drs. Hale and Bennett. In 2001, Florida Hospital became an educational partner with the International Parish Nurse Resource Center and adopted the standardized curriculum for parish nurse preparation. At this point, the approach to congregational instruction was revised, and the Health Ministry Team Building Course was developed. This eight-hour course focuses on health as a congregational ministry and emphasizes the importance of engaging clergy and lay leaders in support of health and wholeness as part of the mission of the congregation. Course participants also receive instruction in the development of an inclusive health ministry team along with strategies for effective health promotion and lifestyle behavior change. More than 350 congregations in central Florida have sent representatives to participate in the health ministry training, and more than 400 nurses from 26 states and Puerto Rico have been educated in the practice of parish/faith community nursing. Health ministry leaders and parish nurse coordinators throughout the United States and as far away as Russia, Australia, and South Africa have used the materials developed by Florida Hospital.

Faith Community Nursing: Scope and Standards of Practice, a document developed by the American Nurses Association with the cooperation and support of the Health Ministries Association, defines faith community nursing as "the specialized practice of professional nursing that focuses on the intentional care of the spirit as part of the process of promoting wholistic health and preventing or minimizing illness in a faith community." It goes on to state, "With an intentional focus on spiritual health, the faith community nurse uses the interventions of education, counseling, advocacy, referral, utilizing resources available to the faith community, and training and supervising volunteers from the faith community" (Health Ministries Association and American Nurses Association 2005).

The document sets forth fifteen standards of faith community nursing practice. The standard of health teaching and health promotion (5B) often presents challenges for nurses coming out of strictly medical settings. Many have had little experience in the field of health science that focuses on the promotion of healthy lifestyles and health behavior change necessary to both manage and reduce the risk of disease. This work includes facilitating presentations that inform congregations on certain health topics. However, to effectively change behavior, efforts must extend beyond health events or presentations. There must be time assigned to identify health risks, followed by the explanation and the meaning of the results. This needs to be accompanied by related health information that can lower the disease risk, individualized and realistic goal setting, and group support for successful health behavior change. An important part of the training program is attention to the standard for collaboration (11) and the standard for research (13).

Recently the Parish Nurse Institute and the Center for Community Health Ministry had an opportunity to study the effect of congregational health education and health promotion activities. With a grant from Winter Park Memorial Hospital, one of the seven Florida Hospital facilities in the greater Orlando area, a three-year project, Project HOPE (Healthy Outcomes through Personal Empowerment) was implemented. This was a demonstration project to measure improvement in health through the work of the congregational health ministry team and the parish nurse in cooperation with the hospital partner. As part of the process, the hospital provided funds to support the part-time salary of the parish nurse and provided health science support for an annual health risk appraisal (including laboratory blood tests, biometrics, and a comprehensive lifestyle questionnaire) and record-keeping to determine baseline health risks and measure participants' health behavior change. Each congregation's health ministry team received an executive summary report indicating prioritized percentages of participants' health needs for the purposes of planning a yearly health initiative. A variety of health and lifestyle change programs were implemented (e.g., nutrition, fitness, weight loss, grief recovery) as well as "train-the-trainer" programs for congregational leaders. The parish nurse's role included developing a health ministry team and responding to expressed health needs for individuals and groups according to the roles of parish/faith community nursing.

Of the 10,732 possible adult participants, 947 chose to participate, with 221 involved for three consecutive years. Eighty were male (75% over the age of 50), and 141 were female (71% over the age of 50). All participants completed a standardized health assessment instrument. The greatest health risks identified were cancer risk (87%), poor nutrition (64%), needing improved fitness (61%), needing weight management (60%), coronary risk (48%), needing cholesterol level management (39%), and needing high blood pressure management (23%).

The outcomes achieved by the end of three years indicated the greatest improvements or risk reductions were in the areas of cholesterol management and nutrition. Other encouraging changes noted were cancer risk reduction and improvement in blood pressure management, weight management, and fitness. Two of the three congregations, convinced of the value of a health ministry, increased the hours of the parish nurse to full-time status and assumed the greater part of the salary by the fourth year—an encouraging sign for the sustainability of the effort.

Interestingly, spiritual health questions were also a part of the measurement process. As one might expect from congregational participants, 99 percent responded affirmatively when asked if their belief in a "higher power" was a source of direction. A series of questions were asked relating to the influence faith has on the participants' meaning and purpose, joy and harmony, comfort during crises, strength to deal with problems, reason to help others, and social contact. Where these questions were concerned, responses such as "yes, very much" and "yes, very often" were in the range of 86–93 percent. The one item that scored lower and indicated a larger potential for improvement was "My faith influences my life as a support and motivation for a healthy lifestyle." Initially, only 69 percent responded "yes, very much" or "yes, very often." By the close of the third year, this percentage had climbed to 79 percent.

Clergy may ask an important question about parish nursing and health ministry: How does health ministry build the kingdom of God, which is the work of the church? The story one Project HOPE participant shared at the time of her second-year health risk appraisal may help answer this question:

> "I can hardly wait for this year's measurement results."
>
> "Why," I asked. "What happened to you?"
>
> She replied, "Last year, I found out that I was at risk, and so I have begun to work on my health. I took a class called Fitness for Life, held here at the church. I learned how to make simple changes—it's not just my diet. It's about a healthier lifestyle. Now my husband and I get up and walk every morning at 5:30. I have lost weight, and I feel great."
>
> Then she added excitedly, "And I am attending church three times a week."
>
> Surprised by this last comment, I asked how often she had attended church before this.
>
> "About once a month," she replied.

Through the work of health ministry and parish nursing, this participant was made aware of certain health risks that, if left unattended, would eventually contribute to poor health or disease. She began facing her situation by acknowledging her personal risk and began to alter her behavior. She attended a class offered by the church, made some simple changes in her lifestyle, altered her diet, and began a reasonable and simple exercise program. She lost weight and noticed that she had more energy, and she proclaimed that she was feeling "great." This participant was affected in positive ways by becoming more engaged in her own health, and she was an influence in her family (her husband joined her in walking). Her new-found "energy" led her to change one other area in her life—participating in her church more. She desired to become more involved in her congregation and had the energy to act on her decision. She wanted to share her experience with someone else: "Let me tell you my story, and it happened here at church."

Also of interest in this work is a "control" congregation that did not have a parish nurse or a health ministry team. This congregation was similar to the others in most respects and open to having a presentation to explain Project HOPE to its leadership and members. In a church of 480 members, 20 participated the first year for baseline data. Each participant was given a personal report. The offer for follow-up health programs was made, but the church did not request any programs or seek further contact with Project HOPE during the year following the initial assessments. When approached to schedule the second year's measurement, there was no response to multiple inquiries and thus no further assessments or programs were arranged. This congregation had dedicated and friendly members, yet without a team of people or a parish nurse to work with the pastor to develop health ministry, the connection between faith and health could not gain traction.

For more information on Project HOPE or to learn more about the Florida Hospital's Parish Nurse Institute and Center for Community Health Ministry, contact Candace Huber, director, at Candace.Huber@flhosp.org, or visit the Web site, www.parishnursing.net.

18

NATIONAL ORGANIZATIONS
AND RESOURCES

There are numerous organizations that have excellent materials and other resources that can be used in planning congregational and community health programs. In this chapter we offer information about some of the ones we have found particularly helpful.

HEALTH MINISTRIES ASSOCIATION

The Health Ministries Association (HMA) is a nonprofit membership organization open to individuals, faith communities, institutions, and organizations. Founded in 1989 as a resource to support faith community nurses (formerly called parish nurses), it has expanded to include program coordinators, lay health ministers, clergy/chaplains, health educators, faculty, and other professionals. The stated purpose of this organization is to encourage and support its members in the development of programs that integrate care of the body, mind, and spirit. The HMA embraces people of diverse faiths, backgrounds, and interests, and currently has more than 1,300 members.

The HMA provides a number of benefits and resources for its members, including an annual conference, online continuing education opportunities, consultation and support, a newsletter, a regularly updated Web site, toolkits and guides, book reviews, discounts on HMA and other conferences, discounts on selected publications, and opportunities for networking.

In addition to participating in the activities and events offered by the national organization, members can join and participate in activities and events offered by regional chapters and HMA networks (e.g., faith community nurses, lay health ministers, clergy/chaplains, etc.). The HMA Web site, open to both members and nonmembers, provides links to faith groups and other organizations that have programs and materials appropriate for congregational health ministries. For more information about the HMA, including how to become a member, you can visit their Web site (www.hmassoc.org) or call 800-280-9919.

Nurses who are interested in learning more about faith community nursing and other individuals who would like more information about health ministries will find the thoughts of Sonja Simpson, a recent president of the HMA, enlightening and inspiring.

I have been involved with health ministry and have been a faith community nurse (FCN) since 1999. It has been the highlight of an interesting and diverse nursing career. Despite my many "mountaintop" experiences in national and state arenas of influence, nothing can take the place of my personal and rich experiences within the arena of health ministry.

Health ministry is a wonderful opportunity for nurses to practice the science and art of nursing. The art of nursing has been greatly diminished by the technology of health care and medical science. Despite the life-saving mechanics of that technology, the art of "holding a hand and fluffing a pillow" has almost disappeared. I believe that true healing is enhanced by a relationship experience—when there is a human connection between the healer and the client. Faith community nursing provides the unique experience for that relationship to occur.

My initial experience with faith community nursing was in Arizona where I lived in a rural area south of Flagstaff and near the beautiful and scenic area of Sedona. I was a volunteer faith community nurse for a small Presbyterian church but soon became the "nurse of the community." I had many referrals from community agencies that heard about and/or experienced, however vicariously, the benefits of a faith community nursing intervention. Most of what I did was case management. Many of my clients were elderly people (upper 70s to 90s) living alone, with family scattered across the country. My ministrations focused on education about their plan of care, nutrition education, "sorting out" medication, and physician visits with the client. Many of the folks did not know how to advocate for their care or what questions to ask or how to tell the physician that they could not afford the medication ordered.

Many of the clients could not be maintained in their home environment, so my job became one of "connecting the dots" for transfer to another level of care. This is a complex process of evaluation of the current situation, financial concerns, and quality of life, and then the appropriate and caring transfer to another level of living. It always involved contacting next of kin and assisting them in the decision-making process of where Mom or Grandma or whoever should go. The mechanics of this care management were always interwoven with concern for the spiritual and "core sense" of the person. Faith community nurses are uniquely prepared and skilled in weaving this complex tapestry of care management.

I was successful in obtaining a small amount of grant funds through the Arizona Community Foundation, which supported my travel and communication needs. By writing the grant, others became aware of the uniqueness of a health ministry program. Within two years, five other churches in the northern part of Arizona developed similar programs.

In 2001, I moved to Grand Island, Nebraska, a medium-sized Midwestern community. I began to pick up the threads of health ministry within my new community and at the same time became networked within the health ministry community on a statewide basis.

I am currently working with a traditional ELCA Lutheran church in developing a health ministry program. The demographics of the congregation indicate that they are largely farmers and families who have been raised generation after generation within that particular church. Women play a very traditional role and seldom exert leadership in marital or family matters.

Several women had questions related to their bodies, aging, nutrition, and exercise. I developed a weekly exercise program for any woman who was interested. It was a joy to teach and to watch individuals improve their balance and agility. The class focused on toning, stretching, breathing, and balance. The ages of the women ranged from the late 50s to the early 80s, with a fourth of the class being in their early 80s. Many women felt that exercise might be too strenuous or that they were not agile enough to do the moves or that they were too self-conscious to exercise with others. I assured them that everyone would work at their own level and that there was no pressure to perform.

As time went on, the women became more engaged and delighted in making *progress. I ended the class about a year ago for reasons not related to the program. After about six months the women asked me to return to teaching because they noticed that their balance and agility had declined without the class. So I reinstituted the class, and I enjoy seeing how much they improve each week. I have incorporated stretch bands and small balls in the class to work on range of motion and body strengthening. The women often lingered after class to ask questions related to their health, and it now has evolved into a post-class coffee and conversation time. I do informal teaching over coffee, which encourages questions. I was amazed at how many did not really understand how their bodies worked and were frustrated with physicians who sometimes seemed to dismiss their concerns—"Oh, you are getting older . . . It is just a part of aging." What I do is give them tips and tools that empower them to do self-care and make subtle changes in their lifestyle and routine.*

I also take monthly blood pressures at this church, which is often like a mini-clinic where the individuals have trust in my listening and advising skills and ask some great questions. Additionally, I teach a monthly interactive class on topics of interest to the group. We laugh and have a good time in the process. Holy friendships occur!

My first exposure to the "big picture" of health ministries came through the Interfaith Health Program, a program funded by a grant from the Centers for Disease Control and Prevention and administered by the School of Public Health at Emory University. It brought together teams from around the country to look at how faith groups can collaborate with community assets such as health systems and public health organizations to improve the overall health of individuals.

I was graced with the opportunity to lead a rural team from Nebraska to participate in the initial training session in 2001. Ten teams from around the country were selected to participate in this new endeavor. It became obvious that both faith communities and health communities are valuable reservoirs of vision, strength, and hope, so it would be natural for them to work together. Individuals who have health issues and emotional concerns often turn to their faith community as their "first avenue of help."

In subsequent years I had the opportunity to lead a national nursing organization focusing on holistic health and to participate in national summits on the connection between faith and health—how healing occurs and how to make health care more humanistic. At the same time, the research on the impact of spirituality on health was becoming more intense and visible, with studies consistently showing that those who have a sense of spiritual identifi-cation have a more successful outcome with their health issues.

During this time, the Health Ministries Association (HMA) was becoming more visible as an organization with a focus on developing the team concept to enhance holistic approaches to care. HMA led the movement to obtain rec-ognition from the American Nurses Association that faith community nursing was a valued and legitimate specialty nursing practice with recognized stan-dards of performance and practice. HMA has become a cherished home for faith community nurses as well as for chaplains, lay health ministers, and oth-ers who focus on intentional care of the spirit as part of their work with indi-viduals and groups facing health challenges. They help clients and other mem-bers of the faith community make connections among themselves and with other resources in the community. As I learned from the Interfaith Health Pro-gram training, the work of others in the Health Ministries Association, and my own experience, the health ministry team weaves a web of relationships, struc-tures, and entities to build a healthier community. If a healthy community is a fabric, then the health ministers and faith community nurses are like the needle to the thread, guiding it back and forth, making it whole.

INTERNET RESOURCES

The Internet is the gateway to endless amounts of information. It's easy to use, accessible, and finds what you are looking for in a matter of seconds. With this in mind, it is no surprise that more and more people are tossing aside books and using the Internet as their main source of information.

There are more than 100,000 health-related Web sites. Keep in mind, however, that since the Internet is a public domain source, anyone can cre-ate a site regardless of their credibility. We recommend that you:

- Use reputable sources. Start with MedlinePlus (medlineplus.gov). MedlinePlus has information that is reliable, current, accurate, mul-tilingual, and written by health professionals. It's free and accessi-ble from any Internet connection.
- Beware of commercial sites. Sites with ".com" at the end of their address are commercial sites whose primary goal is to make a profit, and not necessarily to provide reliable information.

• Check to see if the information is current and accurate. Be sure the information you obtain is written by a health care professional. Look for credentials (i.e., M.D., Ph.D., CRNP, D.D.S., R.N.). Check all information for a date. Information more than five years old is considered outdated.

MedlinePlus (http://medline.gov/)

MedlinePlus is a service of the U.S. National Library of Medicine and the National Institutes of Health. It offers information on more than 700 health topics. These topics are organized both alphabetically and by categories (e.g., Body Location/Systems, Disorders and Conditions, Diagnosis and Therapy, Demographic Groups, and Health and Wellness). For each topic, an overview, the latest news, and links to the Web sites of other federal agencies and health-related organizations are provided. This Web site also has a medical dictionary, an illustrated medical encyclopedia, interactive tutorials, and information on drugs and supplements. Information is provided in Spanish as well as in English. MedlinePlus contains both copyrighted and noncopyrighted material. Noncopyrighted material (e.g., government information at National Library of Medicine Web sites) can be reproduced and copied without permission, but reproductions should contain proper acknowledgment of the source.

Healthfinder.gov (www.healthfinder.gov/)

Healthfinder.gov was developed by the U.S. Department of Health and Human Services together with other federal agencies and is coordinated by the Office of Disease Prevention and Health Promotion and its National Health Information Center. It links to information and Web sites from more than 1,500 health-related organizations. Visitors to this Web site will find a wide range of prevention and wellness topics, a drug interaction checker, and various health-related consumer guides (e.g., Health Insurance, Hospice, Hospitals, Long-term Care, Nursing Homes, Patient Privacy, Public Health Clinics, and Support Groups). Information is provided in Spanish as well as in English.

Healthfinder.gov contains both copyrighted and noncopyrighted material. Noncopyrighted material (e.g., information on the National Cancer

Institute's Web site that was written by government employees) can be reproduced and copied without permission, but proper acknowledgment of the source should be included.

National Institutes of Health (www.nih.gov/)

The National Institutes of Health's Web site offers information on hundreds of consumer health topics. For each topic, it provides links to Web sites that provide information and allow you to download information sheets or brochures that may be reproduced and copied without permission. For example, selecting "Depression" will take you to the Web site for the National Institute of Mental Health, where you will find a 28-page booklet, *Depression,* that can be downloaded and copied. Selecting "Diabetes" will link you to the Web site for National Diabetes Information Clearinghouse (NDIC), a service of the National Institute of Diabetes and Digestive and Kidney Diseases (NIDDK), where you will find a 68-page booklet, *Your Guide to Diabetes: Type 1 and Type 2,* that can be downloaded and copied. This Web site also groups topics under several headings: Men's Health, Minority Health, Seniors' Health, Wellness and Lifestyle, and Women's Health. Many of the Web sites and publications are in Spanish as well as in English.

The National Institutes of Health also has a Web site designed specifically for older adults seeking age-related health information (www.nih seniorhealth.gov). Features of this Web site include a "talking" function that reads the text aloud and special buttons to enlarge the text or turn on high contrast to make the text easy to read.

National Institute on Aging (www.nia.nih.gov/)

The National Institute on Aging (NIA) produces a variety of informational materials on age-related topics for the general public. NIA's AGE PAGES are brief, easy-to-read information sheets (4–8 pages) on topics of interest to older adults or those who live or work with them (e.g., Aging and Your Eyes, Arthritis Advice, Considering Surgery, Diabetes in Older People). NIA also produces lengthier publications on age-related topics (e.g., *Alzheimer's Disease: Unraveling the Mystery, Talking with Your Doctor: A Guide for Older People*) for individuals wanting more extensive information. Both types of publications may be downloaded and copied. NIA also has produced a number of videos that can be purchased for a nominal fee. These can be ordered through the Web site. Many of the informational materials are available in Spanish as well as in English.

Centers for Disease Control and Prevention (www.cdc.gov/)

The Centers for Disease Control and Prevention (CDC), a part of the U.S. Department of Health and Human Services, has as one of its major goals ensuring that people are healthy in every stage of life. As part of its strategy to meet this goal, the CDC provides on its Web site fact sheets and brochures on a number of preventive care measures that can be downloaded and copied (e.g., What YOU Can Do to Prevent Falls, Check for Home Safety: A Home Fall Prevention Checklist for Older Adults, Influenza Vaccine: What You Need to Know). Many of the CDC materials are available in Spanish as well as in English.

National Health Information Center (www.health.gov/nhic/)

The National Health Information Center (NHIC) is a health information referral service established by the Office of Disease Prevention and Health Promotion within the U.S. Department of Health and Human Services. The NHIC Web site provides links to numerous governmental and private health-related organizations. Also available on the NHIC Web site is a comprehensive list of national health observances (e.g., American Stroke Month, National Suicide Prevention Week, National Mammography Day) and an extensive list of toll-free numbers for organizations that provide health-related information, education, and support. Included on this list are organizations that provide crisis intervention (e.g., National Youth Crisis Hotline) and organizations that provide information about rare disorders—disorders that affect less than 1 percent of the population at any given time (e.g., Multiple Sclerosis Association of America).

U.S. Food and Drug Administration (www.fda.gov/)

The Food and Drug Administration (FDA) Web site provides information on medicines (brand-name, generic, and nonprescription), medical devices and procedures (e.g., LASIK eye surgery, mammography, CT scans), food and nutrition, and a number of other health-related topics. Much of the information on the FDA Web site is available in Spanish as well as in English. The information on the FDA Web site is not copyrighted, unless otherwise noted, and it is not necessary to obtain permission from the FDA to republish or reprint noncopyrighted materials. Crediting the FDA as the source of the information is appreciated but not required.

Familydoctor.org
(http://familydoctor.org/online/famdocen/home.html)

Familydoctor.org is a health information Web site sponsored by the American Academy of Family Physicians (AAFP). Topics are organized alphabetically and by a number of categories, including Healthy Living (e.g., Flu Shots, Food and Nutrition), Women (e.g., Breast Cancer, Osteoporosis), Men (e.g., Prostate Cancer, Testicular Cancer), Over-the-Counter Guide (e.g., Pain Relievers, Risks for Special Groups), Smart Patient Guide (e.g., Talking to Your Doctor, Advance Directives), and Seniors (e.g., Arthritis, Memory Loss). The information on this Web site is available in Spanish as well as in English. The content of this site is copyrighted, but information from the site may be printed and distributed if used for nonprofit, educational purposes only. This information should be properly attributed to the AAFP and include a notice of copyright.

AGS Foundation for Health in Aging (www.healthinaging.org/)

The AGS Foundation for Health in Aging (FHA) is a national nonprofit organization established by the American Geriatrics Society. The AGS Foundation serves as a bridge between researchers in aging, geriatricians, and the public. Topics are organized into three categories: How We Age (e.g., The Aging Process, Trends in the Elderly Population), Health Care Decisions and Issues (e.g., Talking to Your Healthcare Providers, Ethical and Legal Issues), and Elder Health at Your Fingertips (e.g., Problems with Joints, Muscles, and Bones; Vision Loss and Other Eye Diseases). Available on this Web site are a number of tip sheets (e.g., Avoiding Overmedication and Harmful Drug Reactions, Cognitive Vitality, Tips for Avoiding Caregiver Burnout) that may be downloaded, copied, and distributed at no charge.

The only stipulation is that they not be altered in any way. Also offered on the FHA Web site is *Eldercare at Home: A Comprehensive Online Guide for Family Caregivers*. This free, 27-chapter guide is authored by more than thirty experts in geriatric care.

My Personal Health Record (www.myphr.com)

My Personal Health Record is provided as a free public service by the American Health Information Management Association, a national non-profit professional association dedicated to the effective management of the personal health information needed to deliver quality health care. The site contains helpful forms that can be downloaded and a step-by-step guide for creating a personal health record. Also on the site is information about how to access your medical records, your privacy rights, and common privacy myths.

IV

APPENDIXES

Congregational Survey

We are interested in organizing some programs on health-related topics that are of interest to members of the congregation. You can help us plan for these programs by completing this brief survey. Please place a check by the topics you would be interested in learning more about.

_____ Adolescent health issues

_____ Alcohol abuse

_____ Anxiety disorders

_____ Arthritis

_____ Assistive devices

_____ Automated external defibrillators (AED)

_____ Cancer

_____ Cardiopulmonary resuscitation (CPR)

_____ Dementia / Alzheimer's disease

_____ Depression

_____ Diabetes

_____ Digestive disorders

_____ Do not resuscitate (DNR) orders

_____ Exercise and health

_____ Eye diseases / vision problems

_____ Heart disease

_____ Hospice care

_____ Hypertension

_____ Living wills / advance directives

_____ Long-term care arrangements

_____ Medications—prescription

_____ Medications—nonprescription

_____ Men's health issues

_____ Mobility equipment

_____ Nutrition and health

_____ Orthopedic problems

_____ Pain management

_____ Palliative care

_____ Prevention of falls and accidents

_____ Respiratory disorders

_____ Respite care programs

_____ Sleep disorders

_____ Smoking cessation programs

_____ Stress management

_____ Support groups

_____ Vaccinations (influenza and pneumonia)

_____ Weight reduction programs and methods

_____ Women's health issues

Suggestions _____

_____

_____

_____

Program Evaluation Form

We would greatly appreciate your taking the time to complete this brief questionnaire. By doing so, you can help us plan for future programs.

I found this program to be informative and helpful.

_____ Strongly agree _____ Agree _____ Disagree _____ Strongly disagree

Based on what I learned in this program, I feel better equipped to handle health matters.

_____ Strongly agree _____ Agree _____ Disagree _____ Strongly disagree

What could have been done to make this program better?

_____

_____

_____

_____

What topic(s) would you like covered in future programs?

_____

_____

_____

_____

Other suggestions or comments?

_____

_____

_____

_____

APPENDIX C

Patient Check Sheet

Name _____ Date _____

How do you rate your health? ___excellent ___ good ___ fair ___ poor
Have you been hospitalized in the last year? ___ no ___ 1 time ___ 2–3 times
___ more than 3 times
Have you used an emergency room in the past year? ___ yes ___ no

Vaccination status (date last received):
Influenza _____
Pneumococcal _____
Tetanus _____

Symptom review (check if a problem):
_____ Visual difficulties
_____ Hearing difficulties
_____ Forgetfulness
_____ Sleeping problems
_____ Depression or loss of interest in usual activities
_____ Other types of emotional distress
_____ Urinary incontinence/leakage
_____ Fecal (bowel movement) incontinence

Have you experienced any of the following events in the last year? (circle answers and describe if yes)

Yes   No   Death of a spouse_____

Yes   No   Death of other close family member_____

Yes   No   Marriage or new companion _____

Yes   No   Change in financial status _____

Yes   No   Change in living situation _____

Yes   No   Loss of long-time pet _____

Yes   No   Divorce or separation _____

Living situation:

_____ House   _____ Apartment   _____ Other

_____ Alone   _____ With other person(s)

List important aspects of your living situation _____

_____

Difficulties with basic and instrumental activities of daily living:

_____ Walking or moving

_____ Using the toilet

_____ Managing medications

_____ Bathing

_____ Personal grooming

_____ Managing money

_____ Shopping

_____ Dressing

_____ Preparing meals

_____ Housekeeping

_____ Transferring (into and out of bed or chair)

_____ Using the telephone

_____ Eating

Patient Information Sheet

Date _____

Name _____ Phone _____

Surrogate decision-maker (and relationship) _____

      Phone _____

Advocate _____

Advance directives _____

Allergies _____

Pharmacy _____ Phone_____

Current Prescribed Medications

Drug	Dosage and Frequency
_____	_____
_____	_____
_____	_____
_____	_____
_____	_____
_____	_____

Current Nonprescription Medications and Nutritional Supplements

_____	_____
_____	_____
_____	_____
_____	_____
_____	_____

Patient needs assistance with these basic and instrumental activities of daily living:

_____

_____

_____

_____

Incontinence problems: Bladder? Yes No   Bowel? Yes No   (circle answer)

Other concerns:

_____

_____

_____

_____

Prioritized problem list:

1. _____
2. _____
3. _____
4. _____
5. _____

Summary Form for Physician Visit

Physician's assessment of overall health status:

_____ Same   _____ Improved   _____ Worsened

New problems identified by physician:

_____

_____

_____

_____

_____

New medications or changes in previous therapy:

_____

_____

_____

_____

_____

Other physicians who need to be seen for consultation:

Name _____

Phone _____

Address _____

Date of appointment _____

Time of appointment _____

Name _____

Phone _____

Address _____

Date of appointment _____

Time of appointment _____

Tests that need to be done before the next visit:

Name of test _____

Location _____

Phone _____

Date of appointment _____

Time of appointment _____

Name of test _____

Location _____

Phone _____

Date of appointment _____

Time of appointment _____

Other instructions: _____

_____

_____

_____

_____

Next appointment (date and time): _____

Reviewed by (physician's initials): _____

Medication Record

Name _____ Date _____ Completed by _____

Primary physician's name _____ Physician's telephone number _____

Prescribed Medication	What Is It For?	Pill Size (e.g., 5 mg, 1 capsule)	Color and Shape	Time Taken (e.g., 8 a.m., 12 noon)	Concerns or Problems	Compliance (e.g., always, sometimes, never)

REFERENCES

Anderson, Gerard. 2007. *Chronic Conditions: Making the Case for Ongoing Care.* www
.fightchronicdisease.org/resources/documents/PFCD_FINAL_PRINT.pdf.
Accessed 6/9/2008.

Baylor University. 2005. *The Baylor Religion Survey,* Waco, TX: Baylor Institute for
Studies of Religion (producer).

Budnitz, D. S., N. Shehab, S. R. Kegler, and C. I. Richards. 2007. Medication usage
leading to emergency department visits for adverse drug events in older
adults. *Annals of Internal Medicine* 147:755–65.

Centers for Disease Control and Prevention. 2007a. What Everyone Should Know
about Flu and the Flu Vaccine. www.cdc.gov/flu/keyfacts.htm. Accessed
6/7/2008.

Centers for Disease Control and Prevention. 2007b. State-Specific Influenza Vaccination Coverage among Adults Aged ≥ 18 Years, United States, 2003–04 and
2005–06 Influenza Seasons. *MMWR Weekly*, 21 September 2007, 56(37);
953–59. www.cdc.gov/mmwr/preview/mmwrhtml/mm5637a1.htm. Accessed
6/8/2008.

Gallup, Alec M., and Frank Newport, eds. 2006. *The Gallup Poll: Public Opinion, 2004.*
Lanham, MD: Rowman & Littlefield Publishers.

Gunderson, Gary. 1997. *Deeply Woven Roots: Improving the Quality of Life in Your
Community.* Minneapolis: Fortress Press.

Hale, W. Daniel, and Richard G. Bennett. 2003. Addressing health needs of an aging
society through medical-religious partnerships: What do clergy and laity
think? *Gerontologist* 43: 925–30.

Health Ministries Association and American Nurses Association. 2005. *Faith Community Nursing: Scope and Standards of Practice.* Silver Spring, MD: American
Nurses Association.

Mace, Nancy L., and Peter V. Rabins. 2006. *The 36-Hour Day: A Family Guide to Caring for People with Alzheimer Disease, Other Dementias, and Memory Loss in
Later Life,* 4th edition. Baltimore: Johns Hopkins University Press.

Miller, William R., and Stephen Rollnick. 2002. *Motivational Interviewing: Preparing
People for Change,* 2nd ed. New York: Guilford Press.

National Institute of Mental Health. 2007. *Depression*. NIH Publication no. 07-3561. www.nimh.nih.gov/health/publications/depression/nimhdepression.pdf.

Partnership to Fight Chronic Disease. 2008. *Almanac of Chronic Disease 2008 Edition: Statistics and Commentary on Chronic Disease and Prevention.*

Pew Forum on Religion and Public Life. 2008. U.S. Religious Landscape Survey. Washington, DC: Pew Forum on Religion and Public Life.

Putnam, Robert D. 2000. *Bowling Alone: The Collapse and Revival of American Community.* New York: Simon & Schuster.

Rabins, Peter V., Constantine G. Lyketsos, and Cynthia D. Steele. 2006. *Practical Dementia Care,* 2nd edition. New York: Oxford University Press.

Rollnick, Stephen, William R. Miller, and Christopher C. Butler. 2008. *Motivational Interviewing in Health Care: Helping Patients Change Behavior.* New York: Guilford Press.

Rosenstock, I. M. 1974. Historical origins of the health belief model. *Health Education Monographs* 2: 328–35.

Statistical Abstract of the United States, 2008. Table 165. Community Hospitals—States: 2000 and 2005. Source: Health Forum, An American Hospital Association Company, Chicago, AHA Hospital Statistics 2007 Edition, and prior years. www.healthforum.com.

U.S. Census Bureau. 2004. U.S. Interim Projections by Age, Sex, Race, and Hispanic Origin. www.census.gov/ipc/www/usinterimproj/. Internet Release Date: March 18, 2004.

U.S. Department of Health and Human Services. 2000. *Healthy People 2010: Understanding and Improving Health,* 2nd ed. Washington, DC: U.S. Government Printing Office.

U.S. Department of Health and Human Services. 2006. *Healthy People 2010 Midcourse Review.* Washington, DC: U.S. Government Printing Office.

Ware, J. E., Jr., and J. Young. 1979. Issues in the conceptualization and measurement of value placed on health. In *Health: What Is It Worth?* ed. S. J. Mushkin and D. W. Dunlop, 141–66. New York: Pergamon Press.

Yearbook of American and Canadian Churches, 2008. Edited by Eileen W. Lindner. Prepared and edited for the National Council of Churches of Christ in the U.S.A. Nashville, TN: Abingdon Press.

SUGGESTED READINGS

Carson, Verna Benner, and Harold G. Koenig. *Parish Nursing: Stories of Service and Care*. Philadelphia: Templeton Foundation Press, 2002.

Chase-Ziolek, Mary. *Health, Healing, and Wholeness: Engaging Congregations in Ministries of Health*. Cleveland: Pilgrim Press, 2005.

Evans, Abigail Rian. *The Healing Church: Practical Programs for Health Ministries*. Cleveland: United Church Press, 1999.

———. *Healing Liturgies for the Seasons of Life*. Louisville, KY: Westminster John Knox Press, 2004.

Gunderson, Gary. *Deeply Woven Roots: Improving the Quality of Life in Your Community*. Minneapolis: Fortress Press, 1997.

———. *Boundary Leaders: Leadership Skills for People of Faith*. Minneapolis: Fortress Press, 2004.

Gunderson, Gary, with Larry Pray. *Leading Causes of Life*. Nashville, TN: Abingdon Press, 2009.

Hale, W. Daniel, and Harold G. Koenig. *Healing Bodies and Souls: A Practical Guide for Congregations*. Minneapolis: Fortress Press, 2003.

Health Ministries Association and American Nurses Association. *Faith Community Nursing: Scope and Standards of Practice*. Silver Spring, MD: American Nurses Association, 2005.

Hickman, Janet S. *Faith Community Nursing*. Philadelphia: Lippincott Williams & Wilkins, 2006.

Jamison, Kay Redfield. *An Unquiet Mind: A Memoir of Moods and Madness*. New York: Vintage Books, 1996.

Koenig, Harold G. *Spirituality in Patient Care: Why, How, When, and What*. Philadelphia: Templeton Foundation Press, 2007.

———. *Medicine, Religion, and Health: Where Science and Spirituality Meet*. West Conshohocken, PA: Templeton Foundation Press, 2008.

Koenig, Harold G., and Douglas M. Lawson, with Malcolm McConnell. *Faith in the Future: Healthcare, Aging, and the Role of Religion*. Philadelphia: Templeton Foundation Press, 2004.

Koenig, Harold G., Michael E. McCullough, and David B. Larson. *Handbook of Religion and Health*. New York: Oxford University Press, 2001.

Mace, Nancy L., and Peter V. Rabins. *The 36-Hour Day: A Family Guide to Caring for People with Alzheimer Disease, Other Dementias, and Memory Loss in Later Life*, 4th edition. Baltimore: Johns Hopkins University Press, 2006.

Manning, Martha. *Undercurrents: A Life beneath the Surface*. New York: Harper-Collins, 1996.

Patterson, Deborah L.. *Health Ministries: A Primer for Clergy and Congregations*. Cleveland: Pilgrim Press, 2007.

Solari-Twadell, Phyllis Ann, and Mary Ann McDermott, eds. *Parish Nursing: Promoting Whole Person Health within Faith Communities*. Thousand Oaks, CA: Sage Publications, 1999.

———. *Parish Nursing: Development, Education, and Administration*. St. Louis: Elsevier Mosby, 2006.

Styron, William. *Darkness Visible: A Memoir of Madness*. New York: Vintage Books, 1992.

The Johns Hopkins White Papers

  Coronary Heart Disease
  Depression and Anxiety
  Diabetes
  Hypertension and Stroke
  Nutrition and Weight Control for Longevity
  Prescription Drugs
  Prostate Disorders
  Digestive Disorders
  Vision
  Back Pain and Osteoporosis
  Memory
  Lung Disorders
  Heart Attack Prevention
  Colon Cancer

www.johnshopkinshealthalerts.com/bookstore

The Johns Hopkins Medical Letter: Health after 50
www.johnshopkinshealthalerts.com/bookstore

INDEX

Richard G. Bennett is a graduate of Dartmouth College and received his medical degree from the Johns Hopkins University School of Medicine. He completed training in internal medicine at Baltimore City Hospitals (now the Johns Hopkins Bayview Medical Center), followed by a fellowship in geriatric medicine. Subsequently, he joined the Johns Hopkins faculty. His work has focused on providing care to older patients, investigating problems common among residents of nursing homes, and teaching the practice of geriatric medicine. For almost a decade, he directed the Fellowship Training Program in geriatric medicine at Johns Hopkins, which is among the largest in the United States. Over the last fifteen years, he has collaborated with Dr. Hale in exploring how health care organizations and religious institutions can work together to improve the health of their communities. Dr. Bennett is the author of more than sixty research articles, reviews, and book chapters. He is currently the Raymond and Anna Lublin Professor in Geriatric Medicine at Johns Hopkins and is the president of Johns Hopkins Bayview Medical Center.

W. Daniel Hale is a graduate of Florida State University and received his Ph.D. in clinical psychology from the University of Massachusetts/Amherst, where he also completed his clinical internship. He served as a clinical psychologist at Orlando Regional Medical Center before joining the faculty of Stetson University, where he is professor of psychology and director of the Community Health Initiative. He has been a consultant to hospitals and mental health centers, and he maintained a psychotherapy practice for more than twenty-five years. In 1992 he began a collaboration with Dr. Bennett that has focused on the development of community-based health programs built around alliances between medical organizations and religious congregations. Dr. Hale is the author (with Harold G. Koenig, M.D.) of *Healing Bodies and Souls: A Practical Guide for Congregations* and numerous research articles on mood disorders, aging, and chronic illness. He has served as president and executive director of the O'Neill Foundation for Community Health since 2003 and is an adjunct associate professor of medicine at the Johns Hopkins University School of Medicine.

3